"As I read Dr. Stern's book, *Grief Connects Us*, it again reminded me of the grief that I have faced both in my practice and personally. Many of us build walls that are impenetrable, but few of us are immune to the power of grief. It is when his sister is diagnosed with cancer and dies followed by the sudden and unexpected death of her husband leaving their teenage sons orphans that Dr. Stern must struggle with grief in the most personal way. By interweaving his own vulnerability and suffering with those of other patients and physicians, he makes us understand that only through empathy and compassion can we truly connect. Powerful, profound, and compelling."

—JAMES R. DOTY, MD, Professor of Neurosurgery and founder of the Center for Compassion and Altruism Research and Education, Stanford University School of Medicine *New York Times* bestselling author of *Into the Magic Shop: A Neurosurgeon's Quest to Discover the Secrets of the Brain and the Mysteries of the Heart*

"In *Grief Connects Us*, Stern dissects the heart-wrenching illnesses of people close to him, and in so doing dismantles the emotional armor those of us in medicine unwittingly don, to accompany his patients in their suffering and feel with them. A transformative read."

—MIKKAEL A. SEKERES, MD, MS, author of *When Blood Breaks Down: Life Lessons from Leukemia* and essayist for the *New York Times*

"Every patient and medical professional who meets the line that separates them will understand when it needs to be dissolved to open the gateway for empathy and compassion. *Grief Connects Us* is an essential guide and inspiration in these challenging times."

—HELEN RIESS, MD, author of *The Empathy Effect,* Associate Professor of Psychiatry, Harvard Medical School

"*Grief Connects Us* is a beautiful book and an important one. The way Dr. Stern writes about illness, hospitals, diagnoses—all the things clouding collective consciousness—from the dual perspective of expertise and lived experience is particularly timely and urgent."

—CATHERINE MAYER, author of *Good Grief* and co-founder of the Women's Equality Party (UK)

grief connects us

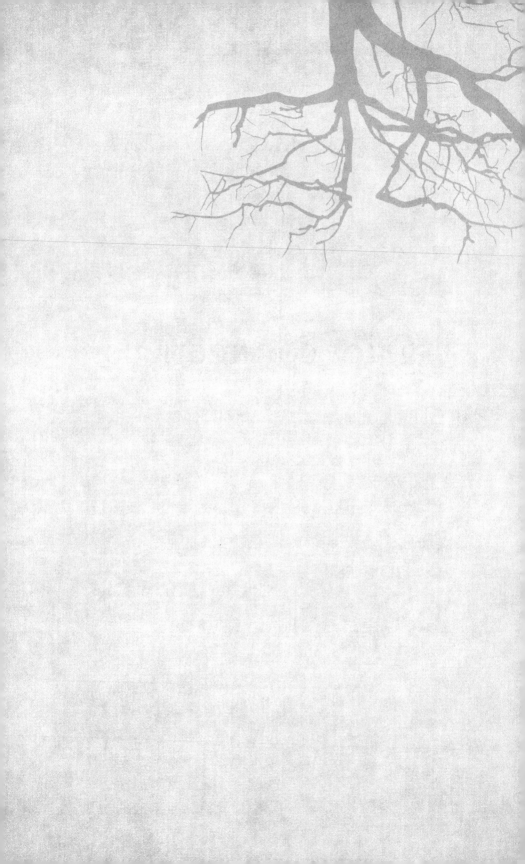

JOSEPH D. STERN, MD

foreword by
Sanjay Gupta, MD

grief connects us

a neurosurgeon's lessons on love, loss, and compassion

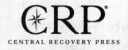

CRP®
CENTRAL RECOVERY PRESS

Las Vegas

Central Recovery Press (CRP) is committed to publishing exceptional materials addressing addiction treatment, recovery, and behavioral healthcare topics.

For more information, visit www.centralrecoverypress.com.

Publisher: Central Recovery Press
3321 N. Buffalo Drive
Las Vegas, NV 89129

26 25 24 23 22 21   1 2 3 4 5

Library of Congress Cataloging-in-Publication Data
Names: Stern, Joseph D., author.
Title: Grief connects us : a neurosurgeon's lessons in love, loss, and
   compassion / Joseph D. Stern ; foreword by Sanjay Gupta, MD.
Identifiers: LCCN 2020041348 (print) | LCCN 2020041349 (ebook) | ISBN
   9781949481518 (jacketed hardcover) | ISBN 9781949481525 (ebook)
Subjects: LCSH: Stern, Joseph D.,--Health. | Neurosurgeons--Biography. |
   Brain--Surgery--Patients--Biography. | Physician and patient. | Patient
   satisfaction.
Classification: LCC RD592.8 .S74 2021 (print) | LCC RD592.8 (ebook) | DDC
   617.4/8092 [B]--dc23
LC record available at https://lccn.loc.gov/2020041348
LC ebook record available at https://lccn.loc.gov/2020041349

Photos are from the author's personal collection.
Photo of Joseph Stern by Aura Marzouk. Used with permission.
Jane Kenyon, "Prognosis" and excerpts from "Chrysanthemums" from Collected Poems. Copyright © 2005 by The Estate of Jane Kenyon. Reprinted with the permission of The Permissions Company, LLC on behalf of Graywolf Press, Minneapolis, Minnesota, graywolfpress.org.

Publisher's Note
This book contains general information about grief, illness and death, and compassion. It examines the impact of cancer and mortal illness on patients, their families, and the physicians who care for them. The information contained herein is not medical advice. This book is not an alternative to medical advice from your doctor or other professional healthcare provider.

Cover design and interior by Marisa Jackson.

FOR

the whelans
Victoria, Pat, Nick, Will

AND

the sterns
Kathryn, Ben, David, Abby

You have all taught me:
The power of love,
That gratitude brings grace,
To live and love large.

table of contents

part three

part four

FOREWORD

by Sanjay Gupta, MD

When Jody Stern first asked me to write the foreword to his book, I really couldn't say no. After all, Jody had been my chief resident when I was just starting my neurosurgical training and even twenty-five years later, I still felt the hierarchal force that compelled junior doctors to automatically follow orders from their seniors. "Yes sir," I responded, secretly wondering where I would find the time. A few months later after the manuscript arrived in the mail, I sat outside one sunny weekend afternoon and read the entire book in a single sitting.

As day turned to dusk, a chill filled the air and the shadows grew long all around me; I was transported into the world of my colleague and friend in a way I had never before seen him. The writing had the familiar cadence and precision expected of a brain surgeon. Few wasted words, a rapid but not rushed pace, and a tidiness associated with the sterility of a well-run operating room. And yet there was something else as well. There was a rawness and a vulnerability not typically seen among our neurosurgical colleagues. There was a venting of compassion and an airing of grief.

It became clear to me that *Grief Connects Us* was not only a book that Dr. Stern wanted to write—it was a book he *needed* to write.

The pain was palpable. Victoria, his kid sister, first became ill with what seemed like the flu, and within a few weeks had taken up residence in an oncology ward. When she died less than a year later, it didn't seem things could get worse for the family she left behind. But then her husband Pat was rendered unconscious after an aneurysm ruptured in his brain without warning. He never woke up, suddenly leaving their teenage boys without parents. The cruelty directed at this family in the prime of their lives was aimless and merciless, and my friend Jody was shaken to his mortal core. It was a reckoning that challenged his identity as a physician and his perceptions of grief and loss as a human. Having counseled so many families through unimaginable loss as a brain surgeon, Jody finally realized that his ability to truly understand and empathize with the anguish of his patients only became fully formed and genuine after he had confronted these painful tragedies on his own.

Over the course of their careers, many doctors develop a sort of emotional armor to help insulate themselves from the overwhelming sadness. For trauma neurosurgeons like us, who often care for patients who are young, healthy, and suddenly dead, that armor can grow thicker and tougher with time. For Jody Stern, his personal heartrending experience revealed just how significant a liability the armor had become, and he set about on what must've seemed a near Sisyphean journey to shed that armor once and for all. This book is the story of that journey, the powerful stories he uncovered along the way, and the very human reactions that bind us together in the face of fear, grief, and failure.

While we are tied together through our shared memories and experiences on this planet, it is grief that connects us most tightly at a near molecular and metaphysical level. Too often we think we must walk that path of grief alone, unwilling or unable to adequately share the depths of our loss. Nothing could be further from the truth. It is here where my friend Jody shines, as he gently holds the hand of the suffering, listens intently, and then weaves the voices of patients and doctors alike into a bold narrative of empathy, compassion, and connection.

We all benefit from a book like this because its greatest currency is the honesty and authenticity of the characters willing to lay bare their soul to help us learn and grow.

AUTHOR'S NOTE

The names of all the patients and families in this book have been changed to avoid violating their confidentiality; however, real names are used in all of the interviews.

a neurosurgeon's journey

My younger sister was an actress. She was creative, trusting, warm, an engaged wife and mother, full of life. Her infectious belly laugh could fill a room. Victoria loved an audience and could keep them spellbound.

I am a neurosurgeon, more comfortable with a single patient in the quiet of an examining room where I can apply logic and science to solve the problems and mysteries of the human body and disease. Through my work, I am educated about mortal illness, having spent more than twenty-five years confronting death and dying.

Had anyone asked, I would have said I believed that my experience as a neurosurgeon insulated me from loss in my own life, that a familiarity with the suffering of others would somehow prepare me for the inevitability of a tragic diagnosis within my own family. I assumed that my proximity to loss enabled me to protect the people I love. And I thought I had a good understanding of what my patients and their families were going through.

When Victoria was diagnosed with leukemia at the age of fifty-one and succumbed to her illness less than a year later, I learned that nothing could be further from the truth. Living through her illness as a brother, rather than as a doctor, has taught me far more about the nature of illness and death than I ever learned in my formal medical training.

In writing *Grief Connects Us* I initially sought to manage my grief over my sister's death, but in the process, I found I wanted to untangle my evolving feelings about death and about the impact that loss has on physicians as well as on patients. I wanted to explore how physicians integrate personal loss into their professional lives, and how these experiences influence the way they relate to patients and their families. I also wanted to better understand the choices patients make and the impact their decisions have on them and on their families.

Physicians are frequently exposed to grave illness, and many of us, such as oncologists, see death every day. We are challenged to function as empathic, supportive physicians, remaining present for our patients through the often confusing and frightening phases of illness, providing advice and counsel yet not coming unglued. In the face of overwhelming loss, doctors must find ways to defend themselves emotionally, but in doing so we often miss the potential for connection and understanding. Some physicians approach their work in a clinical manner, relying on technology or therapies as protective screens between them and their patients. Yet being caught up in the intricacies of a very sick patient's life, sharing time and narratives with them and their families, can lead to pain and regret after a death. How can we maintain connection and not be consumed in the process?

Patients seek empathetic and compassionate connection with their physicians. And, just as physicians do, patients often make decisions out of fear, relying on defensive emotional armor. Like many physicians, I fear failure—of being wrong, of making mistakes, of being overwhelmed by powerful emotions such as grief and sadness I am not sure I can handle. In the process, both patients and physicians miss powerful opportunities for mutual appreciation and understanding. Patients need their wishes to be better understood. They want care rooted in compassion and decision-making framed by the context of their life experiences. Both patients and physicians need to forgo maladaptive emotional armor in favor of a more flexible stance of emotional agility. In the process, they will come to better appreciate each other's unique perspectives.

I used to keep my distance, explaining things thoroughly but often with what I now see as reticence based in my own fear: technically correct, highly verbal, and detached. Now, when I look at myself, I see a little bit of Victoria: I am more demonstrative, more of a friend and a supporter. I try to let my patients and their families know that I care; to pull them close when things are going badly. I try to acknowledge their suffering and also my shortcomings. Through my own experience, a window has opened for me onto the power of solace and nonverbal communication and on the feelings of fear and isolation that come with their absence. Now, I try to keep that window open for others.

Recently, I met a woman who had come to be at her son's bedside in the ICU. He had been in a devastating car accident that broke his neck, tore open his scalp, and shattered his arm and leg. He was not doing well and remained critically ill. We were not sure if he would live or die.

I spoke with Doris about Stephen's injuries, told her how sorry I was that this was happening, and said that no mother should have to go through what she was now facing. I hugged her for quite a while. She cried on my shoulder; I had to wipe away my own tears. The words I shared with her were important, but they only went so far. The hug I offered conveyed as much as, if not more than, all of my words of explanation. In that moment, we became allies. She knew that I knew, and that I was a parent, too; that I recognized her suffering was intense; and that I was trying to acknowledge all she was facing, all that she might lose in this moment of crisis. This made no material difference to the medical facts, nor did it impact her son's care, yet to both of us in that moment it was essential.

Victoria's illness and death broke down the self-protective barriers I had built over the course of my career. As a result, I have come to better grasp the way illness changes our views of our world, often forcing us to reorder our priorities as options narrow. Our perception of time also changes. Any waiting period becomes interminable, as when my sister and I anxiously awaited a doctor's visit or the results of a critical test, whereas momentous events—such as a disastrous and irreversible change in condition—can occur in an instant, often without warning.

While personal and painful, my experiences are far from unique. In reaching out to other physicians and patients, I have been struck by how much we have in common—yet we rarely share these stories of loss, often soldiering through them distressingly alone and disconnected from one another. As physicians, we must shift toward more reasonable expectations of, and care for, ourselves, integrating our personal experiences into our practices and improving the care we deliver to our patients through a system that better accommodates the needs of patients, their families, and the health providers who treat them. As patients, we must insist on meaningful, direct, and honest communication with our physicians, based in compassion and acknowledgment of our personal perspectives. Greater understanding of what we go through will help all of us contend with illness and death in ourselves and those we love, whether we are patients or physicians.

Victoria kept a journal describing her experiences as a leukemia patient and her bone marrow transplant. Her reflections have been threaded throughout *Grief Connects Us*. I also explore the impact of a sudden and catastrophic illness in Victoria's husband, Pat, only eighteen months after she died from leukemia. My own experience of these events led to a series of conversations with physician colleagues and patients whose lives, like mine, have been changed by personal loss and the impact of illness.

I offer specific suggestions for improving the healthcare we deliver to our patients, as well as for dropping the defensive armor we often deploy for self-protection in favor of greater emotional agility. I advocate for earlier and more extensive involvement of palliative care and for reshaping healthcare with compassion as a core value. Within these pages you will also meet two remarkable women, Mary Magrinat and Sally Pagliai, who have grown through their own losses to create a Healing Garden at the Wesley Long Cancer Center, in Greensboro, North Carolina, by restoring an abandoned wetland. This garden is now a refuge that sustains patients and their caregivers, providing their community a green, living place to reflect and find comfort, and linking patients and their families with the natural world.

Finally, I offer some suggestions for how we can improve the way physicians treat both patients and each other. This is my sister's lasting gift: Out of loss comes hope.

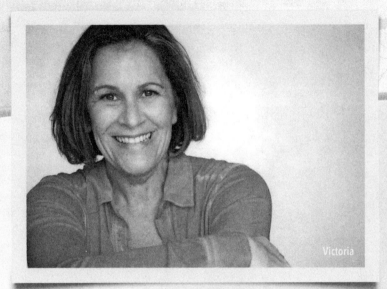

Victoria

Eight months from November 29, 2014 to July 19, 2015 (actually seven months and three weeks if we're being precise, but eight months sounds better):

- 20,131,200 seconds
- 335,520 minutes
- 5,592 hours
- 233 days
- 33 weeks and 2 days.

Four months in the hospital.

Six and a half months away from home.

—VICTORIA'S JOURNAL ENTRY OF JULY 19, 2015

part
one

diagnosis

It started when Victoria developed a flu-like illness that wouldn't go away.

Today marks three weeks and one day since I took up residence at Saint John's.

I arrived on Saturday, November 29, 2014. Pat and the boys were at a USC-Notre Dame game and [were] gone for a long time. Pat had offered to stay home because I hadn't been feeling great for a while, but I encouraged him to go.

For weeks, perhaps months, it felt like my family had been trading every bug, and perhaps we were. Either my body was fighting off too much at once or my immune system was busy elsewhere, so every bug I encountered became a problem. Not sure. Either way, this had been brewing for some time, and it escalated right before Thanksgiving—a time when it was hard to get results, etc.

Earlier that week, I was walking to and from the boys' school, working at Nutrition, and remarked to Anna, the woman operating the cash register to my left, that I wasn't feeling so well. Anna pointed out that I hadn't been feeling well at my last shift two weeks earlier. On my walk home, I found myself very out of breath. I wondered if I perhaps had pneumonia. I'd had walking pneumonia as a kid (I remember fighting coughing fits as I performed on stage in Hamlet at Interlochen one summer), and this felt somewhat familiar, minus the cough.   —DECEMBER 21, 2014

The afternoon of the USC-Notre Dame game, Victoria went out for a short walk and barely made it home. When Pat returned from the game, they went to the hospital, assuming that she had some kind of stubborn flu virus. She had blood work done and was immediately referred to Dr. Fischer, a hematologist-oncologist at Saint John's in Santa Monica, California.

> At first, I went to the ER, where they ran lots of tests. Dr. Fischer had called ahead, so I believe he told them what to check. I was admitted, and then I was moved to a bed on the second floor.
> Turns out Dr. Fischer had them run a flow cytometry test, which showed the presence of a large number of blast cells—abnormal ones you don't want. That's when I got moved to the fourth floor, the oncology unit. Uh-oh. This feeling was echoed a bit when we told Jody, my neurosurgeon brother, about my current state and he replied that he loved me. That made me nervous.   —DECEMBER 21, 2014

The implications of this referral did not initially sink in for her; the fact that disease can transform an active, healthy person into a patient overnight is both disorienting and terrifying, and it would shake Victoria.

My sister was in the middle of her life, managing her identities as wife, mother, actor, writer, and keeper of the master schedule. She was raising two teenage boys, which meant the family's days were filled with carpools, soccer practice, piano and drum lessons, homework, and school activities. Victoria often volunteered at the boys' school, which was within walking distance of their home in Santa Monica.

She was married to a brilliant and devoted man who had weathered two open-heart surgeries, as well as a difficult retinal surgery, in the earlier years of their union. Pat had started his own venture capital business, and they'd endured the stress of some pretty lean years after their move to LA, until his company became a success. Victoria continued to audition and build a creative life beyond acting, writing a screenplay, and producing an award-winning short film. I was always impressed by how they supported each other despite scares and setbacks— and how Victoria still made space to nurture her friends and their budding careers and would always find time for me when I managed to call her.

Our father and our two half-sisters, Madeleine and Alex, were coming to Santa Monica for Thanksgiving. Presumably, Victoria had plans and preparations, but she was too sick to handle them that week. Instead, she found herself in the ER, waiting to be seen.

Her initial blood counts indicated an elevated number of white blood cells with a high percentage of blasts, the immature white cells indicative of a blood-borne cancer. Further testing suggested that she had acute myeloid leukemia, also known as acute myelogenous leukemia.

There are typically two forms of acute leukemia that affect adults, acute myelogenous leukemia (AML) and acute lymphocytic leukemia (ALL). Both derive their names from the types of white blood cells that are being produced in overabundance. In both cases, the immature white cells do not function properly: they can't kill invading bacterial and viral infections, and they choke out the bone marrow production of healthy, normal blood cells, such as red cells, which carry oxygen, and platelets, which promote clotting.

After a repeat blood test confirmed that this was not merely a laboratory error, Victoria had a bone marrow biopsy. This was a "dry tap," which means that the normal marrow has been replaced with so many leukemic cells that there is no longer room for any others. The fact that her marrow was so full of abnormal cells suggested that the leukemia was advanced. My sister was miserable: the overpopulated cells stretch the nerve endings lining the bones, causing deep, aching pain. White blood cells liberate chemicals called cytokines, which cause fevers, explaining the flu-like illness.

The bone marrow biopsy was evaluated by a cytopathologist (an expert in cells), who diagnosed Victoria with AML. The next step was to analyze the genetics of the leukemic cells. The pathologist collected a sample of these cells and assessed the DNA to identify the underlying mutation that had caused the leukemia. This, it turns out, is the most important factor in determining the effectiveness of future treatment and overall survival of the disease.

These tests took more than a week to process. I remember the agonizing wait for results. I had gone from doctor (aware of the waiting time to process tissue samples) to anxious brother—frustrated by the delay, yet powerless to speed up things or even impact her illness. I was distracted and unable to sleep through the night; instead, I would head to my computer, studying graphs and charts and journal articles. If I could learn as much as possible about AML, maybe I could help save my sister.

In the end, Dr. Fischer told me the results over the phone: monosomy 7. We have two copies of each chromosome in every one of our cells. This particular monosomy means that one copy of Victoria's chromosome 7 had been dropped during the copying of the DNA of her white blood cells as they replicated themselves. The loss of an entire chromosome is a big deal with huge implications. From the standpoint of AML, this put her in the worst of all groups of patients with the disease, as monosomy 7 carries a dismal prognosis.

"Promise me you won't research this mutation and check survival rates on the computer," Dr. Fischer cautioned. Hanging up, I rushed to my office and Googled the mutation. It was December, close to my sister's birthday; I stared at the graphs on my screen, wondering if Victoria would live past her fifty-second year.

> What a day. What a thing. I got my hair shaved. Now I look like a cancer patient, in case it wasn't clear enough before. But it does feel better. I am no longer shedding everywhere onto everything, with stray hairs plastered to my pillow, robe, bed, face, neck, and body . . .
> I met with Dr. Siddiqi, who said my induction chemo at Saint John's was a "failure" and that I am to start round two tonight. Very high doses of cytarabine (a.k.a. Ara-C) every twelve hours for four days. Risks include problems with neurological coordination. Thank God Pat is by my side. He makes me feel lucky—even in the midst of this!   —DECEMBER 23, 2014

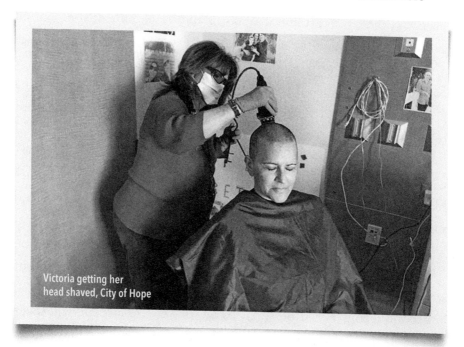

Victoria getting her head shaved, City of Hope

I am still amazed by how quickly one can access information, even about complicated medical concepts and data. I grew up in the era of Medline searches, which involved poring through shelves of bound references. Now all this information is available digitally, so with a few clicks I was able to pull up a staggering amount of material. And none of it was encouraging.

The five-year survival of adult patients diagnosed with AML with the monosomy 7 mutation was 6 percent. This means that ninety-four out of 100 patients were dead within five years. The Kaplan-Meier survival curve (a type of graph that drops toward zero as people die of their disease) had the steepest slope toward zero I had ever seen. The reality is that few people even got close to five years. The prognosis could not have been more bleak.

Yet when I spoke with my sister, she seemed to take this in stride. First, she told me she didn't want to know any statistics. She didn't want to know the survival curve. She was going to beat this illness, and what other people went through didn't matter to her. As we enter the phase of individualized medicine, there is a certain value to this approach. But statistics matter. They inform our decisions and shape our treatment strategies. Insurance often won't pay for treatment without a rational basis.

I felt torn between the numbers I knew and Victoria's desire to be protected from them. She firmly believed that these statistics were not relevant to her and that any deviation from her belief that she would survive somehow diminished the likelihood of success with her therapy, which ranged from the medical approach to alternative approaches like visualization, relaxation therapy, and a focus on nutrition and supplements.

It was hard for me to manage a balance between the information I had and my sister's seeming denial. We were both frightened, but we handled our fears very differently. Her entire focus was on survival and conquering her illness. She said she would accept whatever chemotherapy was suggested and obediently follow the arduous regime prescribed by her doctors. Her path was clear, and her eyes were on the prize: a cure. From the beginning, Victoria did not wish to consider her own mortality.

Early on, it became clear that the only way Victoria might survive was to undergo a bone marrow transplant. She would have to move from Saint John's, a bright, modern hospital close to home, to City of Hope, a hospital on the opposite side of LA dedicated to critically ill patients, with specialties in leukemia and bone marrow transplants. She would also have to say goodbye to Dr. Fischer and meet a whole team of new doctors. Her husband and teenage boys would face a nearly two-hour commute through LA traffic.

The initial plan was to administer a conditioning chemotherapy to beat back the leukemia and then proceed to transplantation. Transplant would allow more aggressive conditioning, or pretransplant preparation, including potent chemotherapy followed by whole-body radiation therapy to kill off her bone marrow (ideally, this would include her leukemic cells), followed by repopulating her bone marrow with the cells of a matched donor. Not only would the donor cells be healthy and free of leukemia, but also—because they were not a perfect match with her cells—there would be a graft-versus-host reaction in which the donor cells recognize the leukemic cells as foreign and attack and kill them.

The problem with graft-versus-host reaction is that the donor cells will also see the body in which they have been placed as foreign and might attack the host's cells and organs, potentially damaging or killing them. One of the tricks of a transplant is allowing graft-versus-host reaction to occur, but not to such an extent that the donor cells ravage the host. This requires antirejection and immunosuppressant drugs to blunt or suppress the immune response of graft-versus-host after the transplant. There would be endless fine-tuning, titrating, and balancing of chemical cocktails within my sister's body.

I began to understand that cancer therapy is a cross between an intricate art form and an elaborate, perplexing chemistry experiment. Each body will have its own unique response, just as each cancer will have its own pernicious character. They will be locked in a battle for survival.

For the first time, I was acutely aware of the degree of terror that patients and their families experience with difficult diagnoses. Up until this point in my life, I believed I had a good grasp on what families were experiencing and knew how to handle physician-family interactions. Now, instead of being in charge of a case, I was the brother of a patient, one of many. I, too, hung on every word from the doctors and medical team, wishing for good news, fearing the bad. The confidence I had known all my working life was evaporating in the glare of my sister's diagnosis, replaced by a profound disquiet that threatened to upend my identity as a doctor.

Victoria always could steal the show. Eighteen months younger than I, she was born with a commanding presence and an innate sense of theatrics. Surveying the scene on her first day of second grade, she announced, with a sweeping gesture of her tiny arm, "Isn't this grand?"

Known at home as "the Imp," my sister delighted in attention and easily inserted herself into the world of towering grown-ups at our parents' parties, climbing from one lap to another. She could be maddening: often our fights would end with me punching her in her arm, after which she would smirk and then run as fast as she could across the house

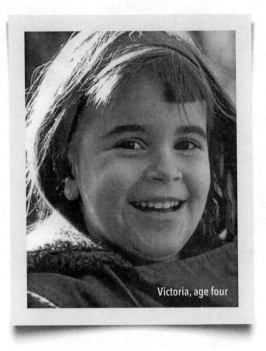

Victoria, age four

to our mother, yelling "Jody hit me!" Only when she was within earshot of our mother would she begin to wail. Inevitably, this worked. Mother would drop what she was doing and envelop Victoria, suddenly dry-eyed and smiling from ear to ear, in a protective embrace, chastising me for hurting her "baby." I resented the con, yet I had to admire Victoria's skill.

I also admired her energy and enthusiasm, and gladly followed as she took on adventures I was far too timid to attempt on my own. She would talk back to neighborhood boys far bigger than she, always willing to take on any dare or challenge they tossed her way.

We lived in Washington, DC, with our parents and our older sister, Caroline, in a rambling house overlooking a wooded ravine. Victoria and I had the run of our leafy, affluent neighborhood—for the most part— free of adult supervision. In a thick bamboo patch, we dug pits and hideouts with some of the older boys on the block. Only years later did I realize that we were acting out Walter Cronkite's CBS nightly news, recreating firefights and ambushes between the North Vietnamese and US soldiers. Most of the boys were older, and Victoria and I watched, excited yet afraid, as they dug trenches and traps for the other kids to fall into.

Victoria was fearless in a way that Caroline and I were not. She could also be dramatic, and sometimes it was impossible for a sibling to tell the difference between drama and trouble. I remember the night she was driven to the hospital after our parents found her choking and gasping for air, having somehow put her head through the sleeve hole of her pajamas. At the time, I couldn't tell if she was truly hurt or whether she was just basking in the attention; I was suspicious of the whole thing. Still, she had little bruises over her eyes and a puffy face for days, so it couldn't all have been for show.

Our father had been an attorney on the Warren Commission after clerking for Earl Warren, and we grew up amid dinner-table discussions and speculation about the assassination of President Kennedy. After his time on the Commission, our father returned to his partnership in a DC law firm.

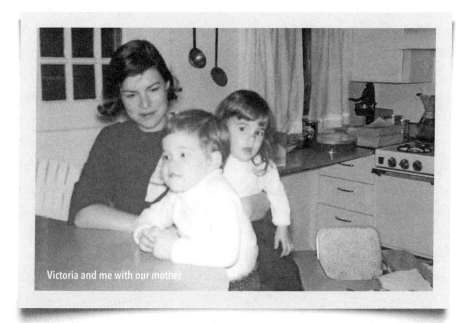

Victoria and me with our mother

Our parents frequently entertained with boisterous dinner parties, and after our bedtime, Victoria and I crept to the stairs to spy on the revelers on the floor below as they argued politics and occasionally sang around the piano. One evening we watched, fascinated, as a drunken guest sprawled out on the living room couch, singing loudly. Despite our gymnastic efforts to work our necks over the railing for a better view, we could only see the back of his head. And one time, Tom Lehrer came to our house. Victoria and I stood in rapt attention, as we were big fans of "Vatican Rag" and "New Math."

Victoria and I were nine and eleven, respectively, when our family moved to London. We'd expected to stay two years, but just as our sojourn was meant to end, our parents announced that they were getting a divorce and planned to stay on for another year. With the family adrift, my sunny, precocious sister became my only anchor. Caroline was unhappy and wanted to return to the States, so our parents sent her to a boarding school at home. Now fast allies in an uncertain world, Victoria and I remained in London.

We moved with our mother to a small mews near Kensington High Street and our father relocated to a house of his own in Notting Hill, where we spent occasional weekends. Meals with our father were awkward, full of prolonged silences and disconnected small talk, and the food was often appallingly bad: clumped spaghetti with canned tomato sauce; overcooked broiled spareribs; Chinese takeout. Sometimes we walked sullenly together down the street to Giles for fish and chips. It was reassuring to have Victoria with me for the obligatory family moments we endured. At each visit, we surreptitiously inspected the bathroom, looking for evidence of new "visitors." Our mother dated some as well, and we were merciless in our imitations of her boyfriends, including one who had a wandering eye—Victoria, with practice, was able to make her eye do the same thing.

Despite our divided family and households, and our older sister's departure, Victoria and I, both now teenagers, fell in love with our new independence. London was full of protests and hippies, pop art and

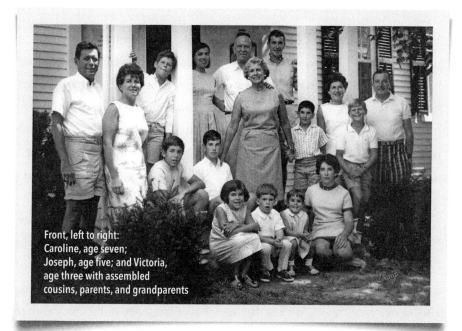

Front, left to right:
Caroline, age seven;
Joseph, age five; and Victoria,
age three with assembled
cousins, parents, and grandparents

music. For two teenagers with time to kill, everything seemed possible. We listened to music and wandered around Kensington High Street and Notting Hill Gate, mostly on our own. We adopted cool new wardrobes of velour tops, clogs, and brushed-denim trousers. In an effort to fit in with the other kids, we began to smoke cigarettes and professed a willingness to try beer and alcohol, which led to a lot of repressed nausea and the development of acting skills, as we enthusiastically pretended that we liked the bitter taste.

Victoria's companionship gave me the courage to explore. Some of my fondest memories of our time in London are of Saturday mornings on Portobello Road. A discerning antique-buyer's paradise, it was also a candy store of possibilities for kids with no discernment whatsoever. There was adventure in picking through piles of junk to find treasures. The dealers rented out stalls in cramped, narrow passageways behind the storefronts. They kept their goods in boxes piled on rickety wooden tables, and if you engaged them in a chat, you got a history lesson in family crests or sword fighting or how to properly set a formal table. After the World

Wars, many of the grand estates in England became unaffordable for the titled class, so the titled had unloaded family possessions for the rest of the world to harvest: boxes of tarnished silver overflowing with delicate teaspoons and grape scissors, enormous soup spoons, and knives with flat ivory handles; colored glass goblets; umbrella stands made from the legs of elephants; gold pocket watches; and stately grandfather clocks with intricate brass hands. Strange, slightly menacing, porcelain figures piled on rickety tables dared you to pick them up. I generally didn't; Victoria often did.

I admired rows of miniature lead soldiers from various regiments: splendidly dressed Prussians; Russian Cossacks on horseback; British World War I infantrymen, their uniforms exact replicas down to each beret and lapel ribbon. Meanwhile, Victoria paraded around the stalls with a wide grin on her face, trying on fox fur stoles like the ones our grandmother Liboo wore back in Chicago. Victoria commanded attention, but also forbearance, as her performances generally amused, rather than annoyed, the onlookers. Everyone was in on Victoria's jokes; they were never at anyone else's expense. Surrounded by lead armies, I watched from a safe distance—mortified by her theatricality, yet envious of her confidence. In my memory, Victoria is always there with me on those rainy winter mornings, trying on hats adorned with exotic feathers and sorting through trays of rings set with gaudy gemstones, each one bigger than the next.

During the school holidays, we traveled together by train. Our parents arranged for us to stay on a farm in Brittany so we could learn French, presumably through immersion. This learning experience turned out to involve hauling rocks from the host farmer's fields and watching in complete horror as he castrated a bull. We attended an outdoors camp in Wales where we learned to pitch a tent and rock climb. Most of our holidays occurred in the spitting rain, and while I took to the outdoors and continued to seek adventures in the mountains and trails, I think my sister learned to appreciate a nice hotel with hot running water and "creature comforts." I am pretty sure she never went camping again.

As one extra year became two, reflecting the uncertainty of our situation, Victoria grew interested in theater and began performing in school productions. I took to science and crew at my all-boys' school.

Caroline commuted back and forth from the States each summer and for the longer school holidays. My sisters missed each other and made an effort to keep in touch, eleven-year-old Victoria's letters already suggesting her grown-up self:

Dear Caroline,
I'm sorry that you feel that way about me. I really don't want you to dislike me, which I feel you do.

I miss you so much, and I really wish you were not angry with me this summer.

I don't have as many boyfriends as everyone makes out, just I'm always falling in love with people, but they don't always feel the same way about me.

Well, I hope your view of me will change, but I cannot do anything to change it for you.

I was so upset about the day I saw you, because it wasn't long enough, I barely saw you.

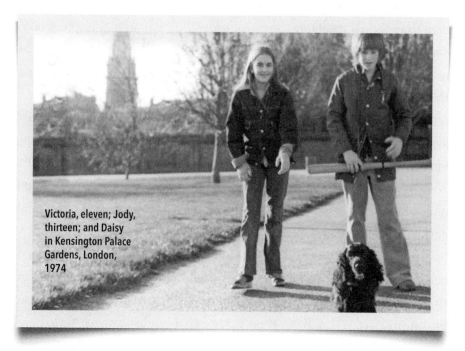

Victoria, eleven; Jody, thirteen; and Daisy in Kensington Palace Gardens, London, 1974

Well . . .
Jody has started judo and I'm very scared about being practiced on.
Mommy is working very hard, and I think it is leading to success.
Dad and J are fine. I am just about to go out to dinner with him . . .

XXXX

Our father bought a canary yellow E-Type Jaguar, and on Sunday afternoons Victoria and I went out on the roads with him. My father drove with the convertible top down, seemingly oblivious to the risks, both his children standing up in the back and holding onto the front seats, wind ripping through our hair as we sped along the M40 at over one hundred miles an hour. I don't believe we ever considered the use of seat belts. I felt safe with my sister, and none of my childhood would have been as thrilling without her wholehearted embrace of adventures large and small.

When Paul McCartney was trying to obtain a visa to return to the United States in the hopes of a Beatles reunion, our father served briefly as his lawyer. Marijuana charges stood in his way; despite Dad's efforts, McCartney's entry was forbidden. One of my fondest memories was being invited to the Hammersmith Odeon to attend a Wings concert. This was the heyday of theatrical 1970s rock, and we had landed right in the thick of the action. Victoria and I found the deafening noise and flashing lights electrifying. Our balcony seats were with VIPs, and we spent the evening running around collecting autographs from the famous audience. The list included Roger Daltrey, Eric Clapton, Gary Glitter, Suzi Quatro, David Frost, and Ringo Starr and his wife Barbara Bach. Some of them were completely drunk, and all of them were happy to sign our concert posters. We were giddy with excitement and, once again, entirely unsupervised.

Afterward, we met Paul, Linda, and the other members of Wings and got them to sign our posters as well. I would never have had the courage to ask them for their autographs—Victoria didn't hesitate. Not the least bit intimidated, she walked right up to her intended targets, thrust out her poster, and requested their signatures. My poster was signed as well, but only after Victoria had staked her claim.

When Victoria was thirteen and I was fifteen, we returned to DC and the quiet, nurturing campus at Sidwell Friends School. She jumped back into life with all of her old friends; it was as if she had never left.

Both our mother and our father eventually remarried other people. I graduated from Sidwell and went to the University of Michigan-Ann Arbor, where I studied liberal arts and majored in history. When I later decided to attend medical school, I stayed at Michigan for medical training and then for neurosurgical residency.

Victoria graduated two years behind me and went on to Smith College. She starred in many school productions, only some of which I saw, and performed in summer stock at the Weston Playhouse in Vermont, later moving to New York to begin her stage career in earnest. In the city, she shared a cramped Upper West Side apartment with her friend Monique from Smith. Clothes, costumes, and leather boots cluttered the floor and filled their one (red velvet) couch. To me, visiting from the disciplined world of surgical residency training, it seemed like an impossible way to live. Even using their bathroom was often the cause of great embarrassment for a brother, festooned as it was with lingerie draped over wire hangers. Tubes of makeup occupied every spare surface.

My sister had a greater tolerance for risk and rejection than I ever did. She would audition for parts over and over, only to be passed up, yet she would return the next day and try again. I would have found that degree of exposure intolerable. I was drawn to the more clearly defined life of a surgical resident. It didn't require the same leap of faith, despite the long hours and demands. If you successfully completed the training program, you would be qualified to practice as a neurosurgeon. The direction, the expectations, were clear. In many ways, mine was the easier path.

Acting, by contrast, is risky and unpredictable. Victoria's optimism and confidence helped her weather countless rejections without losing her self-esteem or passion for acting. She was innovative, and often daring. Always determined, she took the initiative: when she couldn't get a part, she went about making her own movies. She supported her fellow actors, cheering their successes and consoling them when they failed.

Victoria loved being in New York, loved the energy of the city. She worked as a waitress most evenings, auditioning and attending theatrical workshops during the day. It was during these years that she was introduced to the man she would eventually marry.

Pat was starting his own venture capital firm and Victoria was trying to establish herself as an actress. At some point, they decided that her acting prospects would be better in Los Angeles and Pat's business ventures could be just as successful there as they were in New York. Flying by the seat of their pants, they packed up their belongings and moved across the country to begin a new life.

Once Victoria became ill, I realized, looking back, how easy it was for us to take each other for granted. How easy it was for me to take her for granted. My time and attention were consumed by work and by family, by all the scheduled activities of soccer tournaments, ballet, tennis matches, and bar mitzvah preparations. My sister and I lived parallel lives on opposite coasts with children at different developmental stages, immersed in different activities. We spoke infrequently. I felt I had been neglectful. I felt guilty that we had become so removed from each other's lives. Part of my fear when she received her diagnosis was that too much time had passed and too great a distance had grown. Would we be able to reconnect? As it turned out, over the course of her illness one of my great pleasures was the discovery that those connections were still very strong and very much alive for both of us—and that, with my medical training, I could be truly helpful to Victoria in her time of crisis. Later, I learned from her journal that these feelings were mutual.

I am so glad Jody is here. Not only is he here to give me his wise advice and council [sic] but also I am really enjoying my time with him. He has been our go-to consultant throughout. Pat and I have called him repeatedly to help us decipher various medical pronouncements. And, when he is not here, he texts me daily to ask how my numbers are. He has been very much part of our team. And now that he is here again, I'm able to enjoy spending time with him. With him living in North Carolina, raising three kids, and leading the busy life of a neurosurgeon, we haven't seen each other nearly enough. I feel like we are making up for lost time, having wonderful talks about so many things. He is also just sitting with me, as Pat has done, keeping me company, hour after hour. The mask and gloves don't bother him much since he is used to wearing them for work. He has played a lot of games with me, too. It has been a real treat to have him here with me, keeping me on this side of sane.   —APRIL 20, 2015

learning to tie knots/ the arc of a career

The arc of a neurosurgical career is like a surgery to remove a brain tumor or an AVM [arteriovenous malformation]. In the beginning, you are very aggressive and bold. Early on, the tumor is not near any critical structures. But, as the case progresses, you become more and more timid, until at the end, you become fearful.

The trickiest part of the surgery is at the end, when you remove the last part of the tumor, which is wrapped around the carotid artery or the optic nerve.

And that is when you know you can hurt a patient.

—KYLE CABBELL, FELLOW TRAINEE AND CURRENT PARTNER

Stocky, with thinning sandy hair and head perpetually tipped in a quizzical way, Dr. Julian "Buz" Hoff was a remarkable teacher, researcher, surgeon, and leader. He was the chairman of the Section, now the Department of Neurosurgery, at the University of Michigan. He was also the reason I became a neurosurgeon. Equipped with a seemingly limitless supply of aphorisms, which he delivered with impeccable timing, he made us laugh. He also cut the tension. "I'll have you farting in silk pajamas," he would announce at a particularly arduous moment in a surgery. Or he'd lean over with a conspiratorial wink and declare, "You haven't had this much fun since the day the pigs ate your baby brother."

Dr. Hoff inspired devotion and hard work by example, bringing kindness, compassion, and humility, as well as superb skill, to the practice and teaching of neurosurgery. He was a true mensch and treated his patients and staff with dignity and respect. He was devoted to his patients and they to him—so much so that they would often confide they were doing well rather than complain, because they didn't want to disappoint him.

He understood the importance of keeping one's cool and not getting caught up in the moment. I remember running down the hall of the hospital during my second year of residency to inform him about a patient who was deteriorating from a hemorrhage he had had in his brain.

"Doctor Hoff!" I blurted out. "We have a problem."

He stopped me and looked me in the eye, suddenly serious. "No, the patient has a problem. You and I are just fine." Buz was restoring calm and order, defusing a tense situation, maintaining perspective—all essential skills of an effective physician. He was pointing out the importance of being concerned and invested, but at the same time maintaining awareness of the distinction between the patient and the doctor and not becoming overwhelmed by the drama of the moment.

It is an awesome thing we are entrusted to do to people. We cut their skulls open, reroute blood vessels, remove tumors from deep within their brains, rebuild their spines with rods and screws, and replace disintegrated bone with artificial discs. There is an awful lot to master on the way to becoming a fully competent independent neurosurgeon. It takes seven or eight years of post-medical school training to acquire the skills needed to practice general neurosurgery.

There were only two residents in each training year, and we were all encouraged to work as a team. Cooperation and mutual support were crucial. I completed my training before work restrictions came into

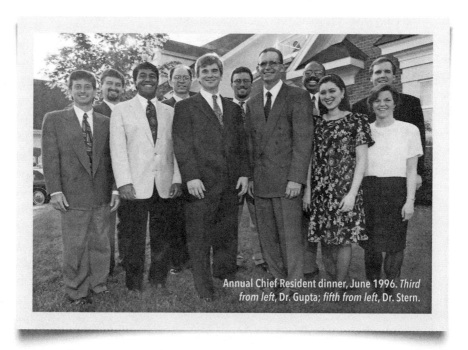

Annual Chief Resident dinner, June 1996. *Third from left*, Dr. Gupta; *fifth from left*, Dr. Stern.

effect after the Libby Zion case, when 100-hour-plus workweeks were the norm, rather than the exception. Yet despite the long hours, the spirit of collegiality permeated our training. There were nine professors in addition to Dr. Hoff in the Department of Neurosurgery. They all shared a dedication to teaching, reinforcing the humanity of the program. Each resident worked closely with an attending surgeon, one-on-one, in the operating rooms, where the attending directly inculcated skills and techniques to the neurosurgeon in training.

Neurosurgery training programs are notoriously grueling. They begin with a yearlong general surgery internship, followed by six more years of neurosurgery residency in a teaching hospital. The load of responsibility and complexity of the surgeries increase with each training year, until you are performing the most difficult cases largely on your own by the end of the seventh, otherwise known as the Chief Year. We began our apprenticeship with fairly routine lower back surgeries and gradually made our way up the spine to the neck, the skull base, and finally the brain.

29

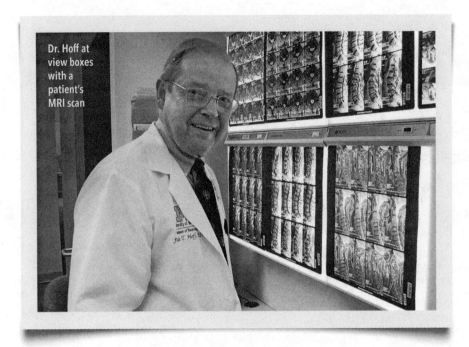

Dr. Hoff at view boxes with a patient's MRI scan

There was also much to learn about the operating rooms themselves. At the University of Michigan there would often be as many as ten or twelve people in each operating room, including the attending surgeon, resident trainees, medical students, scrub technicians, nurses, and the anesthesiologists and their trainees. Technicians would shoot X-rays, operate specialized equipment such as lasers, nerve monitors, and ultrasound imaging, or manage extensive trays of implantable hardware if we were performing spinal reconstructive surgery. Not infrequently, the neurosurgeons would work with teams from other medical disciplines, such as otologists (for acoustic or skull-base tumors) or general or vascular surgeons to perform unusual surgical exposures, such as temporarily moving large blood vessels to allow us access to the front of the spine for our surgeries.

The training is demanding and thorough. On completion of residency, you have developed a unique set of skills and judgments, as well as the flexibility to incorporate new skills and techniques going forward.

Even twenty-five years ago, we neurosurgery residents were taught

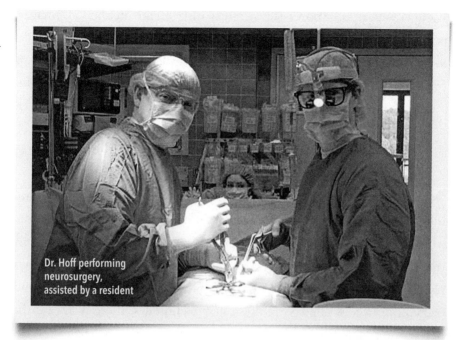

Dr. Hoff performing neurosurgery, assisted by a resident

how to integrate new technology into our operating rooms and to function as a cohesive group. A good neurosurgeon (or any good doctor, for that matter) is a lifelong learner. Many of the surgeries we now perform regularly had not even been conceived of during the years of my formal residency training. Often, we improve the way we operate while in practice, continually adjusting our surgical techniques as new approaches become available. For example, all of the minimally invasive spinal surgeries have come about in recent years, replacing older operations that had wider exposures. We now perform extreme lateral decompressions of nerves that have become pinched by bones, ligaments, or ruptured discs and fusions in the lumbar spine through tubular retractors, which we pass through the patient's side to dock onto the disc space, navigating with X-rays and electrical monitoring. We place screws in the spine over wires placed through stab incisions based on X-rays. None of these techniques existed during my formal training.

I recently performed an operation on the base of a patient's skull and upper cervical spine using intraoperative CT scanning and a navigation system that superimposes the surgical instrument on the CT images, making for a safer, more accurate surgery. These navigation systems didn't exist during my training. Now, when I place a screw into the first cervical vertebra, I watch the computer monitor as well as the patient, seeing a virtual projection of the screw to confirm that it will be well positioned in the bone and not penetrate the vertebral artery, which courses millimeters away. The slightest injury to this artery could mean disaster for the patient.

The most recent innovation introduced to the operating room involves the use of robots to place spinal hardware. I can only imagine what will come next. As surgeons, we evaluate the technologies and master them on cadavers before incorporating them into our practices, always trying to balance the goals of increasing safety, improving outcomes, and decreasing risk. While trying these new techniques, there is always the potential of increased risk to the patient, particularly in the early stages of adoption.

Through the process of training, you change, taking on greater and greater responsibilities. You reach a level of familiarity and confidence with the details of your specialty so that complex tasks become routine. Yet no matter how routine the work becomes, you still bear the weight of responsibility for patients and the sacred trust they place in you to bring them through illnesses or surgeries without complications or disability.

One of the most sobering transitions in my career came when I finished my residency program and took on the role of attending physician. No longer was I reporting to a chief resident or a professor. I had become directly responsible to my patients. With this daunting privilege came an unfamiliar, almost palpable weight. As a resident, I would arrive in surgery knowing the patient's case and our plan of treatment. We operated as a team, and even in my seventh year an experienced professor was always by my side, guiding and advising me. During my training, I did not meet with the patient or the family before the surgery. I did not counsel the patient about other options, and I rarely saw the patient again after his or her hospitalization. My duty was to learn how to operate on the person in front of me, honing my skills and learning protocols, procedures, and diseases. This helped distance me from the feelings of sadness and guilt I now experience if I cannot relieve the suffering of my patients, if I cannot cure their disease, or worse yet, if I cause them injury.

There were many reasons why my fellow residents and I respected Dr. Hoff so much, but one of the biggest was that he was willing to have tough conversations with patients and to admit when we had failed. He was scrupulously honest and did not shirk responsibility. Now that I am practicing on my own, this is even more striking to me: Dr. Hoff accepted ownership of errors that he did not actually commit but that were those of his trainees, me included. He understood this to be an inherent part of the training process. Other attending doctors would go out of their way to avoid these uncomfortable moments with patients and their families; Dr. Hoff embraced them, seemingly without flinching, as part of his role.

The responsibility we shoulder as surgeons can be immense. One of my colleagues once said, "No matter how many great operations we perform, we are only as good as our last surgery." Others say, "If you aren't having any complications, then you aren't doing enough surgery." Some doctors protect themselves by shunning genuine connection with their patients in the first place, but most care deeply and take very seriously the trust placed in them. It is hard to promise to care for your patient, promoting yourself as the best choice to help him or her with his or her problem and outlining the plan of treatment, and then fall short in the delivery. Many times, the failure may not be a technical error but an unanticipated bad outcome, such as an intraoperative aneurysm rupture or bleeding following a surgery. The implications may be dire and can even lead to a patient's death. The sense of personal responsibility, and often of failure, after a bad outcome is no less when a technical error is not the underlying cause; you experience a sinking feeling, often accompanied by nausea, even when rationally you know that everything went as planned during the operation.

I have watched new graduates enter practice and experience for the first time what it means to be "on your own" in the operating theater, making grave decisions and having to stand by them. Even when a technically demanding procedure is performed beautifully, a patient may develop an unanticipated complication. Most surgeons are devastated by such a result. They had done everything correctly, and skillfully executed the latest technique, but still the patient had done poorly. In that instance, it is hard for us to reassure ourselves with all the *good* results we had and not agonize over the permanent change and disability an individual patient may experience under our care. No longer was there an attending physician to carry, or at least share, the burden. It is ours alone.

Complications occur with regularity and are unpredictable. They haunt and shape doctors. We dream about them and remember them always. Facing them and our patients is crucial. Admitting, accepting, and ultimately forgiving our failures is an essential part of becoming a healthy, mature, and effective neurosurgeon. Swathing ourselves in arrogance and dishonesty or avoidance doesn't work. I learned by example from Dr. Hoff, but it has taken me the better part of my career to sort this out for myself. Still, one of the hardest parts of my job continues to be exposing my patients to risk and managing and accepting any suffering I may have inadvertently caused them.

Not only is the transition from trainee to attending sobering within the context of medical errors and complications, the burden we face caring for patients with life-threatening illnesses such as cancer is eye-opening. As a resident, I was fascinated with the anatomy of brain tumors and the technical aspects of surgically removing them. Performing the surgeries and caring for the patients immediately before and after their operations was more than a full-time job, and I lacked any understanding of the longitudinal care required. Now, when I meet a person with a newly diagnosed brain tumor, I will follow my patient for the duration of his or her illness, from diagnosis to surgery, to postoperative care, to chemotherapy or radiation therapy (if necessary), through possible recurrences, and potentially to deterioration and death.

This is an entirely different experience from that of the brash, youthful trainee participating in complicated surgeries peppered with potential risk to the patient, but without any long-term relationships with the patient and the patient's family. Despite our intense knowledge of neurosurgical procedures, as practitioners we leave our teaching programs with little training in counseling our patients about their illnesses or in how to negotiate the decisions we need to make with them as they confront life-altering and, occasionally, life-ending illnesses. Even as we become highly competent in the operating theater, we still bear the weight of responsibility for bringing our patients through illnesses or surgeries without complications or disability.

The problem is, no matter how good we are, complications are inevitable, often taking us by surprise. The other day, I performed a fairly routine surgery to decompress a man's cervical spinal cord, which was under severe pressure from arthritic bones and discs; he was rapidly losing the use of his hands and the ability to walk. I performed this surgery with one of my newest partners, and together we did what we thought was a careful and meticulous job.

My patient woke up after the surgery barely able to use his legs, with his right arm weaker than it had been before he was put under anesthesia. I have replayed the entire surgery in my head numerous times and am not sure what, if anything, I did wrong. This is scary, since I do not know what I would do differently in the future; thus, it is not clear how I would prevent the same outcome. Ultimately, this is one of the greatest burdens of being a neurosurgeon: the sometimes unforeseeable and inexplicable bad results and grave complications, along with the awareness that these complications can reoccur and that despite the best of intentions, preparations, and practice, they will hang across your shoulders like a great heavy coat.

Fortunately, these cases are rare, but that does not make them any less agonizing for me or the other people involved. Over time, this particular patient will likely recover function and regain independence, but he will never be his normal self again. I know that the surgery was the right thing to do, since he was losing his motor skills, and that the situation was almost certain to worsen without treatment. But this knowledge doesn't begin to relieve the sense of failure I feel—that all surgeons feel—when things do not go according to plan and patients are injured in the process.

One of the advantages I have gained from longer-term connections with patients is the chance to witness truly remarkable recoveries, which can only be fully appreciated with the passage of time. I have cared for many young victims of car accidents who were comatose in intensive care for weeks on end, often with invasive monitors in their brains, tracheostomies and feeding tubes placed surgically, and eventually transferred for rehabilitation. I have seen them come back months later, walking on their own two feet back into my office, breathing and eating normally, scars healed, returned to their preinjury selves. This perspective is a source of inspiration and wonder. The medical teams who only observe the patients during their acute hospitalizations do not often see these stunning transformations. One of the greatest rewards for me is to be there for these moments with my patients.

Physicians experience remarkable victories as well as devastating losses. The former are the stories that keep us going. Sometimes we are able to save people, occasionally in spectacular fashion.

One day after a snowstorm, about five years into my practice, a trauma doctor notified me of the arrival of a "level 1 trauma," indicative of life-threatening injuries. I rushed to the emergency room to find Paul, a teenage boy, bleeding profusely from his scalp. He had been intubated with a breathing tube and was being wheeled into the CT scanner. The scan showed an open depressed skull fracture. A large piece of the top of his skull had been driven into his brain, cutting the sagittal sinus, the head's principal draining blood vessel. We raced Paul's gurney up to the neurosurgical operating room and unwrapped his head. Blood was pouring out, soaking the sheets. After a rudimentary shave, I prepped his scalp with betadine and began to operate. With a scalpel, we opened the scalp laceration further, elevated the depressed bone fragments, and repaired the venous branches into the sagittal sinus. We ligated, or closed off, the sinus in front of the lacerated portion of this blood vessel with a heavy silk suture. The anesthesiologist gave the boy multiple units of blood as we performed the repair. We were eventually able to control the bleeding, and then reassembled his skull like a jigsaw puzzle with titanium plates and screws. He spent a day asleep on the ventilator in the ICU, and the next morning we allowed him to wake up.

Paul's parents spent a sleepless night in the ICU waiting to understand the results of their son's injuries. We learned that this seventeen-year-old was their only child. His high school had been closed for a snow day. He had been riding on an inner tube, towed by his friend's car across the fresh snow of a farmer's field. The boys did not realize that the fence along the edge of the field was made of concrete posts designed to look like wood. The inner tube shot to the side in a wide arc as the car turned sharply. It gathered speed and launched Paul headlong into one of the concrete posts. His school friends called an ambulance and he was rushed to the hospital.

After we lightened the sedation and removed his breathing tube, we were all relieved to discover that Paul was responding appropriately, indicating his brain had not been badly damaged. He healed rapidly from his physical injuries, went to rehabilitation for several weeks, and was later discharged home. Early on, he had some cognitive impairment and problems with impulsive behaviors, but eventually he made a full recovery. He ended up missing a semester of high school, but he graduated the next year. Able to attend North Carolina State University, he later became an engineer. I took him back to surgery just before he went to college and rebuilt his forehead with an acrylic resin to smooth the remaining, still-noticeable defects in his skull. He is now happily married, and a father. Paul has gone on to build a meaningful life of his own. His accident will eventually become a footnote in that life, or a story he will tell his children, rather than a defining moment, or worse, someone else's tale of a life that ended before it had fully begun.

An important element of our training that prepares us for our later careers occurs through immersion in neurosurgical diseases, from which we gain a sense of context that helps define our expectations and shapes our interactions with our patients. We come to see progress in patients where many others do not. Following commands in the ICU often means that patients will hold up two fingers when asked to do so. Other doctors will joke that this is "normal" only for a neurosurgeon. But, over time, a patient who has gone from a noncommunicative coma to following simple commands represents enormous progress.

I remember, during my training, telling my wife about a young girl in the hospital with a brain tumor who was making progress each day. We struck up a friendship. I would play cards with her on her bed if I had a few spare minutes. After several weeks, I brought Kathryn in to meet the girl. My wife was shocked. Where I saw daily progress, she saw a sick child—face bloated from high-dose steroids and head shorn, a stark red incision on her scalp—who was severely affected by her cancer. My norms and expectations had been reset by daily exposure to Kaitlin's disease, whereas for Kathryn this was an unfamiliar and frightening landscape far from her normal experiences.

Paradoxically, as we neurosurgeons move through our careers, we gain a clearer understanding of the risks involved in our profession. New doctors push the envelope and are eager to try complex and daring procedures—embracing risk, driven by a sense of infallibility and youthful optimism. Often, they are oblivious to the vulnerabilities of a patient, likely because they do not feel vulnerable themselves. I see this in my three young adult children, and while I admire their belief that everything usually works out and that almost anything is possible, this attitude is both a virtue and a curse, particularly in the operating room. As we age, we sense greater frailty in ourselves, often tempered by the accumulation of our own losses, both personal and professional. There is growing awareness that what we do is inherently dangerous and full of risk.

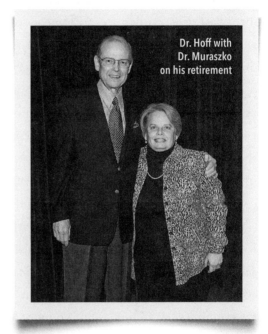

Dr. Hoff with Dr. Muraszko on his retirement

I had already been practicing in Greensboro for ten years when Dr. Hoff retired from the practice of neurosurgery, after he developed acute leukemia. He and his wife were traveling in Italy when he became ill. They flew back to Michigan. He died eight months later. In addition to being chairman of the Department of Neurosurgery at the University of Michigan for twenty-five years, he had trained over fifty neurosurgical residents who are currently in practice throughout the United States, many of whom attended his memorial service on a beautiful spring day in Ann Arbor.

Some of his former residents conjectured afterward that his leukemia was the result of radiation exposure he'd received early in his training.

Little was understood then about the long-term effects of radiation exposure. Trainees used to perform direct carotid arterial punctures without lead shielding for arteriography (now we use catheters placed in the patient's groin or wrist, and stand behind lead-lined windows when X-ray images are being taken). These tests were done routinely to assess for brain shift; the X-rays showed displacement due to blood clots or tumors of the arteries feeding the brain prior to surgery. Now these direct arterial studies are no longer done, replaced later by CT scans and then later still by MRI (magnetic resonance imaging). At the time of Buz's early training, however, decisions to operate were made based on these direct punctures and skull X-rays. An entire field of radiology, assessing "square shift, round shift, pineal shift" by interpreting skull films, has been supplanted by newer imaging modalities. Today, even the more sophisticated angiography methods have been largely replaced by noninvasive imaging studies as neurosurgery and its practitioners continue to adapt to new techniques and knowledge.

The line separating me from my patients is becoming less distinct as I age. I remember my eagerness, in training, to operate on patients with rare, fascinating brain tumors. The patients were often in their fifties and sixties, which to someone in his twenties seemed a lifetime away. Many of my patients now are my age or younger. I realize that it is luck or chance that has spared me some of the fates I've witnessed, and I know that in time, I will become a patient myself, just as my sister did.

part two

the patient's perspective

> ... Over days the IVs came out,
> And freedom came back to him—
> Walking, shaving, sitting in a chair.
> The most ordinary gestures seemed
> Cause for celebration ...
> —JANE KENYON, *CHRYSANTHEMUMS*

> Some people come in your life as blessings.
> Some come in your life as lessons.
> —MOTHER TERESA

With Victoria's leukemia, I saw that I had vastly underestimated the extent of the anxiety, fear, and helplessness patients and their families experience when confronting catastrophic illness. I had always been able to maintain a certain detachment. Although invested in and connected with my patients, I kept myself sufficiently removed to be able to perform surgery on them without becoming overwhelmed. This is a difficult course to navigate in the best of circumstances, but with my sister in the hospital I found myself increasingly distracted by her plight. I was speaking with Victoria each day, discussing her situation and reviewing her blood counts with her, yet the physical distance between us felt too great. At work, I began to perceive my patients' concerns through my sister's eyes. Suddenly, I was much more aware of the depths of their fear and suffering. I began to doubt myself.

An oncologist friend of mine, Gus Magrinat (interviewed in Chapter Eight), used to joke with me about the absurdity of a shrinking violet neurosurgeon. People want a confident neurosurgeon, not someone who is unsure of what he or she is doing. It takes tremendous confidence to advise a patient to have brain or spinal surgery and to advocate yourself as the surgeon. I often struggle with the expectations I place on myself, as well as with what is reasonable for patients to expect of me. Since there is no such thing as a perfect surgery (everything can always be done better), the promise of perfection is not realistic. But now the corrosive feelings of doubt were less about my abilities to perform surgery and more the result of a greater sense of empathy and identification I was feeling toward my patients. Loss of detachment can be a problem for a surgeon (this is one reason many medical students opt not to go into surgery in the first place), but some distance is necessary in order to concentrate on the technical aspects of procedures and get the patient safely through an operation.

At City of Hope, I was a brother trying to support his sister, attempting to comfort her and to interpret the medical facts for our family. If I felt this as a trained physician, how were people without an intimate understanding of the world of medicine able to cope with these issues? Or was my knowledge and training actually getting in my way? Was it perhaps better to take my sister's approach and not ask hard questions?

Soon after Victoria's diagnosis, I saw William E. Williams (interviewed in Chapter Nine), a thirty-six-year-old African American man with a newly diagnosed brain tumor, in my clinic. William was a delightful person with whom I developed an immediate rapport. A musician and gospel singer who played in his local church ensemble and traveled frequently with his pastor, he had been perfectly healthy until he had a seizure and lost consciousness while on the road. His friend rushed him to the emergency room at Moses Cone Hospital in Greensboro, where an MRI scan showed a brain tumor, most likely a low-grade glioma, or intrinsic brain tumor, which takes origin from the glial cells, the supporting framework that feeds and provides structure for the neurons of the brain. The emergency room physician started William on Levetiracetam, a drug to prevent seizures, and he had no further seizures for a week. He came to my office to discuss his situation. He was calm and trusting, but clearly terrified. William's father accompanied him. The elder Mr. Williams peppered me with questions.

I explained that William would need a craniotomy, or surgical opening of the skull, to remove the tumor as completely as possible. This would be his best chance of long-term survival. Depending on how aggressive the tumor appeared to the pathologist, who would determine its grade or severity, further treatment might include follow-up imaging with MRI scans at regular intervals and possibly chemotherapy or radiation therapy, or both. After more discussion, William agreed to have the surgery. We planned to go ahead with it the following week.

Prior to surgery, we obtained an additional planning MRI, which allowed us to create a three-dimensional model of William's brain using our navigation computer in order to reference our precise location during the operation. This is important in most brain surgeries, but particularly so with low-grade gliomas, since the tumor is often indistinguishable from the normal surrounding brain. Without this tool, it would be impossible to define adequate borders of a complete surgical resection.

The marriage of advanced technology and neurosurgery has allowed greater precision in removing tumors, also making possible smaller openings in the skull. While I was having my discussion with William, I was picturing Victoria: newly diagnosed, scared to death, putting on a brave face, and trusting her doctors with her life. Just as William was afraid for his own life, she was terrified that she might die. I became aware of a certain audacity—an audacity bordering on hubris, in fact—

in my suggestion to William that he needed to have the top of his skull opened up and that I was the man to do it.

Detachment is an essential component of my job. As a doctor, I would not have been able to treat my sister. My judgment would be affected and I would make poor decisions, based more on emotion and less on professional opinion. While I cared about William, he was my patient and not a beloved member of my family. And I was glad for that separation. I had always walked comfortably inside the rarefied world shared by physician and patient, shielded by what radiation oncologist Matt Manning (interviewed in Chapter Eight) refers to as "emotional armor." This armor allows doctors to continue working despite the many tragedies in the lives of those we encounter. If we are consumed by the fear and grief our patients and their families experience, we can no longer help them. Our challenge is to care, to empathize, to honestly appraise the effectiveness of our treatments (ideally with data, rather than anecdotally), and to learn from our mistakes. We must continually improve the way we care for our patients without becoming overwhelmed by this daunting task.

My wife once asked me if being a surgeon felt like being a pilot. I see a crucial distinction: while both professions demand attention to safety and intimate knowledge of specific complex systems, in a plane crash the pilot dies, too. In surgery, if disaster strikes, the patient dies but the surgeon and the surgical team remain intact. There are clear limits to empathy. As Dr. Hoff said often, "We do not have a problem. It is the patient who has a problem." At the end of the day, I walk away from a patient's suffering and his disease. But when it's a family member lying in the hospital bed, there is not as clear a separation. When we ourselves become patients, that safe distance ceases to exist. While we may not be flying the plane at that point, we are definitely on board.

During the time I was treating William, everything about my work felt more difficult, and the weight of my responsibility became heavier. For the first time I was experiencing the acute awareness of surgery's inherent dangers that comes as one reaches a high level of skill and technical accomplishment. Victoria's illness was causing me to see more clearly the suffering and risks my patients were experiencing, matters I had previously blocked from my mind.

William's surgery went extremely well from a technical standpoint. I took out the entire tumor, confirmed the next day on an MRI. The tumor was long and cylindrical, extending below the motor cortex of the supplementary motor area, an area in front of the motor strip, into the motor control areas of his brain, which controlled his right leg movements. When William awoke from surgery, he had perfectly intact sensation but was unable to budge his leg at all. Later, the weakness began to improve and became confined to his foot. We took him for an emergency CT, which showed there was no evidence of stroke or bleeding at the surgical site. Over the course of months, William would completely recover his leg strength, but at the time I did not know what to expect. On top of this, the pathologist informed me that the tumor was not grade two, as we had hoped, but a higher grade of three. This carried a considerably worse prognosis and required both radiation therapy and chemotherapy, in addition to regular visits with a neuro-oncologist.

Sitting in the small examining room in my office, I told William that his diagnosis wasn't good. At the same time, I was thinking about my sister, about the pieces of bad news her doctors were compelled to dole out after each test result came back. I now understood what it must feel like to be on the other side. It was sobering and frightening. I fought back tears as I discussed what this tumor would likely mean to William, who was about to get married and had plans for a family of his own. I also told him what was going on with my sister. That afternoon I booked a flight to Los Angeles.

At first, Pat was upset with me. He had carefully organized visitors to their home and to my sister at City of Hope. The timing of my visit would disrupt that schedule. Still, Victoria wanted me to come, and I was able to take the time off, so we went ahead with this new plan. The gravity of

Victoria's illness was clear; I felt a desperate need to see her. I had gone from daily communication with Dr. Fischer to nonresponsiveness from Victoria's new doctors. Normally, physicians will speak with family members who are physicians to keep them updated on a patient's prognosis, but the new doctors were not responding to my calls and messages.

Our family was trying, without great success, to identify potential bone marrow donors. My older sister, Caroline, and I had arranged for DNA testing for HLA typing and were awaiting the results. In the meantime, Victoria's sample was tested against the database of potential donors. The test had produced only one potential match out of twenty-two million.

The process of learning about HLA testing and bone marrow registries opened entire new worlds to me. I learned about altruism in the Jewish world, through organizations such as Gift of Life. I learned that the Holocaust partly explains why it is hard for people of Jewish heritage to find matches. Because the Nazis eliminated six million Jews, many potential descendants who could have become donors simply do not exist. I had not realized how directly tied to ethnicity HLA typing is, although this makes sense. People are more likely to find potential donors from within their tribe or ethnic group, just as they are more likely to find matches from among siblings and immediate family members.

I also learned how timing is everything. Victoria became ill around Thanksgiving, which meant that the search for potential donors was interrupted by the Christmas and New Year's holidays, a time when databases were difficult to access and charitable organizations were closed for up to two weeks. The prolonged waits added to the sense of anxiety and urgency surrounding Victoria's illness.

Leukemia was not Victoria's first cancer diagnosis, but her third. She had been diagnosed with amelanotic melanoma about five years earlier after a mole on her neck appeared to grow and was removed surgically. Melanoma frequently looks black with the pigment of melanin, but a small subgroup of melanomas lose their pigment and are white. They can spread throughout the body but may appear discolored. This process of losing previous features can occur with cancer and is often why tracing the source of a malignancy can be difficult.

While the margins of the original resection were not clear (melanoma tends to spread to the rest of the body after invading locally through the layers of skin to the blood supply, which is deep in the surface layer), Victoria underwent regular surveillance studies that showed no evidence of new melanoma tumors.

A few years later, she was diagnosed with thyroid cancer. After discussions with an endocrinologist and a surgeon, she elected to have this mass removed. It was a difficult decision, as the general course of thyroid cancer can be slow, but in the face of a previous malignancy she became convinced it was the safe, appropriate choice. Both of these procedures were relatively straightforward, although the regulation of her thyroid function with replacement hormones proved imperfect and, at times, frustrating.

Not surprisingly, these diagnoses created a heightened fear of cancer in my sister. Victoria became vigilant about her health and that of her family. She read about diet and wellness, ate wisely, exercised regularly, and practiced yoga. She believed that her lifestyle would safeguard her against future cancers.

It is not uncommon for people to develop multiple, seemingly unrelated malignancies or for cancer to run in families. Understanding of the genetics of cancer is improving rapidly as we identify genetic predispositions. Our DNA has built-in mechanisms to correct mutations and prevent cells from multiplying out of control. Tumor suppressor genes such as p53 are part of the normal cellular machinery to halt the development of malignancies. Our cells are programmed to reproduce and to die in an orderly fashion. We have two copies of each gene as a safety mechanism, so if one is damaged the second will override this malfunction and continue to function properly. But if a person already has a mutation in one of the p53 genes, then another insult to the person's DNA, such as a mutation like the loss of a chromosome, can lead to loss of normal cellular function and the subsequent growth of a tumor.

Most of the time, these malignancies occur in patterns. Seemingly unrelated cancers are in fact related through damaged tumor suppressor genes. Some patients will develop multiple endocrine neoplasias, while some women will develop breast or ovarian cancer. There are also families with high rates of cancer in which another mutation, *BRCA*, associated with high rates of ovarian and breast cancers, is passed to female offspring.

But Victoria was not a member of any of these cancer families. Other than our grandmothers, who developed malignancies at advanced ages, no one in our immediate family has had cancer. The three types Victoria had are not typically associated with each other; thyroid and pancreatic cancer go together, but melanoma, thyroid cancer, and leukemia do not. It was a perplexing trio of diseases that did not raise alarms because there was no known relationship between these separate cancers. A recent population study suggests that leukemia rates are consistent with random mutations, rather than the result of some inherited genetic propensity to developing leukemia. Victoria's cancer history could be merely "bad luck." Still, three malignancies in a relatively short period did not seem likely to be the product of random chance.

Immediately after receiving the diagnosis, Victoria became obsessed with tumor suppressor genes and seeking an explanation for "why me." I tried to explain p53 and some of the other things I knew about the genetics of cancer, but also—and most importantly—I told her about the limitations of our current state of knowledge about the disease. She was worried that if she had a genetic propensity to cancer, she might have passed it to her sons and that they would be at risk for developing malignancies as well. No conclusive tests currently exist to answer this question, but even if they did, it is unlikely that they could lead to prevention or early treatment. Later, as my sister adjusted to the new reality of leukemia, these questions seemed to recede in their urgency, although throughout her illness she was consumed by the desire to protect her children, both by preventing illness in them and by conquering her blood cancer and remaining available to them as their mother.

It was the beginning of 2015. Victoria had been in the hospital continuously, first at Saint John's and later at City of Hope, since Thanksgiving. She had initially received conditioning chemotherapy through Dr. Fischer at Saint John's, but when it became clear that she would need to undergo a bone marrow transplant, he transferred her to the care of Dr. Margaret O'Donnell, a leukemia and bone marrow transplant specialist at City of Hope.

Victoria and her family had gone from a close-to-home facility with a warm and accessible physician and staff to a specialty cancer hospital east of Los Angeles in the foothills of the San Bernardino Mountains. While everyone was helpful and efficient, this place felt much more like an institution.

My sister was placed in a special HEPA-filtration room because her white blood count was dropping to dangerously low levels and she had to avoid exposure to other people and their germs. Everyone had to gown, glove, and put on a special filtration mask before entering. The isolating effects of her disease were hitting home. Some days, Victoria was allowed to walk in the halls, but only when her white blood count was at an acceptable level. When it was low, along with her ANC (absolute neutrophil count), she was restricted to her room and visitors were kept to a minimum. Her days were often long and lonely.

I arrived in Los Angeles in early January. The plan was for me to stay with Victoria out near Duarte and give Pat a week of respite. Their boys needed to get back into the post-holiday school routine and adapt to having their mother away for long stretches. Pat had been driving to City of Hope from Santa Monica each morning, a trip that, depending on traffic, could take anywhere from one to three hours. He would spend the day at the hospital before driving home to have dinner with Nick and Will and get them to bed. Our immediate family and several of Pat's siblings had rotated in and out of the Whelan household, while friends organized meals and carpools. The gravity of Victoria's condition was sinking in. Pat began to recognize that this would be a long, arduous fight for her life.

After several weeks of commuting, Pat rented a small house in Monrovia, a short drive from City of Hope. I spent the week with my sister in her hospital room, sleeping at the rental house each night. At the end of my visit, I drove back to their home in Santa Monica and stayed with my nephews while Pat returned to Victoria's bedside. I had spent little time on LA freeways and found the experience incredibly stressful, connecting between six highways each way to get between Santa Monica and Duarte. I knew we were fortunate to have the resources to manage this arrangement. I also knew that Victoria was lucky to have been admitted to a hospital specializing in leukemia to which she did not have to travel (many people had to come from out of state to be treated at City of Hope). I was reminded of how many issues the majority of my patients juggle while they put their lives on hold to battle illness or care for a sick family member. Through it all, they must figure out how to manage bills, prescriptions, childcare, and missed work.

Before I'd arrived, I'd called to speak with Dr. O'Donnell or her treating physician. I left a message but never received a call back. This went on for several days. My sister did not understand the treatment plan and anxiously awaited a meeting with Dr. O'Donnell to discuss the team's strategy.

Meanwhile, Caroline and I submitted cheek swabs to see if we qualified as potential bone marrow donors and waited for the results. Victoria was receiving chemotherapy to kill the blast cells (immature white cells), but the drugs were also destroying other blood components, including red cells and platelets. The plan was to give her a round of chemotherapy followed by a bone marrow biopsy to see if the blasts had disappeared. They would allow her a week or so to recover (and possibly let her go home) and then repeat another round of chemotherapy, followed by a second bone marrow biopsy. In an attempt to kill off her bone marrow, the second round of chemotherapy would be even stronger, followed by four days of whole-body radiation therapy. The course of treatment was a brutal assault on Victoria's body, but she had no choice. If she did nothing, the leukemic blasts would take over and she would probably not survive more than a few months.

Once the bone marrow is destroyed, the patient, without an infusion of new stem cells, will die. The whole process is precarious and time sensitive; you bring the patient to brink of death and then try to revive him or her with the transplanted stem cells. Even with donor-matched cells, there is a period of high risk prior to "engraftment," when the new cells take hold. This is a crucial time when the recipient is susceptible to potentially fatal infections or other problems, such as internal bleeding.

The donor cells, even though they are close to a perfect match, will still identify the cells of the recipient as foreign and, therefore, a threat. Without strong drugs to suppress the body's immunity, these donor cells will attack the recipient's organs and try to kill them off—a graft-versus-host reaction. This can prove fatal. The drugs that suppress the immune response leave the patient vulnerable to infection by bacteria, viruses, or fungi, making the need for isolation that much greater.

Because of their susceptibility to infection, transplant patients are not allowed to leave the hospital. And even after they stabilize following transplant, they must stay nearby so they can be rushed back in the event of sudden illness. Even though Victoria had only come from across Los Angeles, her transplant team felt the distance would be too far to go if she became ill. Therefore, she was required to stay on the grounds of the hospital, or at least within a few minutes' drive, for the first hundred days after her transplant.

I wanted to meet the doctors and establish the timeline for treatment. With Dr. Fischer, I had been able to speak candidly about the severity of Victoria's leukemia, and we both acknowledged the unfavorable odds. At City of Hope, it was difficult to develop allegiances with my sister's team of doctors. They were overwhelmingly busy, acutely aware of the precariousness of each patient's condition, ordering and analyzing dozens of blood tests, trying to fine-tune each treatment. With leukemia and bone marrow transplants, timing is everything. The hospital relied heavily on the nurses to reassure and educate the families of their patients. I was grateful for their compassion and willingness to answer my sister's questions. Most of the time this was helpful, but occasionally some of the explanations were confusing and added to Victoria's sense of foreboding and anxiety. I began to see that while the hospital represented hope and great medical advances, it was also a place where people came to die.

reconnecting/
first visit

There is no profit in curing the body if, in the process, we destroy the soul.
—SAMUEL H. GOLTER, AN EARLY LEADER OF CITY OF HOPE

I arrived at City of Hope for the first time on a sunny, mild Saturday and set about gathering information on my sister's case. One of the hematology fellows on duty informed me that no decisions would be made until Dr. O'Donnell returned on Monday. Fortunately, the nurses dedicated to the care of my sister were very supportive. Many of them commute hours to work at City of Hope and feel a passionate commitment to their patients and to the mission of the hospital. I came to appreciate nursing care in a whole new light; the nurses were our lifeline and spent hours tending to my sister in her room. They changed and maintained her IV lines, and helped her to the bathroom and occasionally to the shower; they constantly tended to her beeping IVs and pumps, which delivered intravenous medications. Attuned to my sister's physical and emotional needs, they were readily available and caring, often making encouraging comments that helped to relieve moments of despondency, quell Victoria's anxiety, and bridge the long gaps between visits from her doctors.

City of Hope's research and clinical buildings are sprinkled over the grounds, surrounded by gorgeous gardens. Victoria's room was in the tallest building, Helford, where most clinical care is administered.

As I got off the elevator, I was struck by how empty the hospital seemed. There was no one in the waiting area or in any of the hallways leading to my sister's room, apart from occasional personnel. I was used to the hustle and bustle of the hospital at home, with families filling the patient hallways, carrying flowers, and talking on their cell phones. There was a large window at the end of the waiting area, and below I could see the lush green gardens and flowering trees. Inside, all the doors to the patients' rooms were closed.

Even though the world of hospitals is familiar to me, I felt afraid as I headed toward my sister's room. A nurse had apprised me of the strict protocol and visitation rules. I was not permitted to hug or even to touch Victoria. I had tried to prepare myself emotionally, but I didn't know what to expect. Would she look terrible? Would her pallor or frailty frighten me? I felt driven to see her, but at the same time I was apprehensive about what she would be like. I knew that she had lost all her hair and color. Would she still seem like my sister, or would she seem like "a cancer patient"? I felt like a foreigner in a strange hospital, a doctor who understood the systems in place to care for patients, yet without any connection to the medical or nursing staff to make me feel relevant.

I knocked on her door, washed my hands at the sink outside her room, and donned a mask, gown, and gloves from a cabinet above the sink, just as I would do when scrubbing for surgery. When I entered her room, my dread and foreboding were replaced with a surge of relief. Victoria seemed full of energy, with the same buoyant optimism that had seen us through the tumultuous London years. She was bored by the lack of human contact and the sterile environment, but otherwise she was the same sister I had always known and loved. While any physical contact was strictly forbidden, I could tell that she shared my sense of relief. I looked right through the hospital setting and equipment to Victoria, bald, in a hospital gown, and wrapped in blankets, but still projecting warmth, with the same wry, mischievous smile she always had.

The years of separation dissolved. With so much common history,

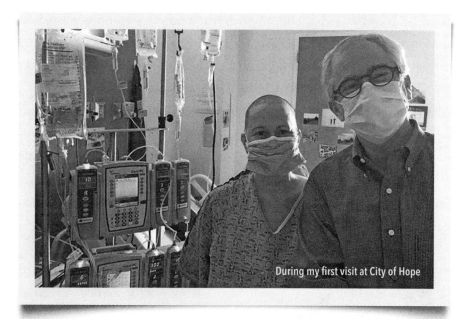

During my first visit at City of Hope

we didn't need to explain ourselves. Just being together felt reassuring. Victoria had decorated her room with large pictures of Nick and Will, photos of Pat, and a family portrait of the four of them on the beach in Santa Monica. Adding a personal touch to her otherwise antiseptic

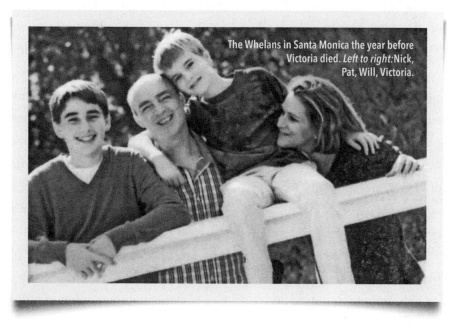

The Whelans in Santa Monica the year before Victoria died. *Left to right:* Nick, Pat, Will, Victoria.

hospital room was challenging given the many restrictions placed on patients with severely compromised white blood cell counts. Visitors were limited to a few friends and family members, and we were not allowed to bring living things like flowers or plants. Simple activities, like walking in the hall, were prohibited. While Victoria could look out onto the gardens below, even cracking open her window was forbidden.

She had lost most of her hair, including her eyebrows. Normally immaculately coiffed, my sister had tired of the bald patches and itchiness and asked the hospital beautician to shave her head. She lost her appetite, eating sparingly because of her nausea.

A large whiteboard on the wall across from Victoria's bed served as a focal point and spelled out the various blood draws, procedures, and maintenance schedule for the day.

Phone numbers for family contacts were inscribed in the upper corner of the whiteboard, along with the names of her doctors, medical team, nurses, and aides. Below them, posted in blue marker, were her recent laboratory results. On any given day, she might get a transfusion of platelets. This was done when her platelet count fell below 20,000. The normal range for platelets is 150,000 to 300,000. Without platelets, you are at risk of spontaneous bleeding from the gums or nose, and you can also bleed internally into your organs or brain. The chemotherapy had wiped hers out, but transfused platelets do not last as long as your own, so the number had to be checked each day. Victoria's daily regime was a balancing act, and her body's individual responses to the assaults of chemotherapy and radiation were still unknown. We had entered a new world of blood counts; even small changes seemed significant and could bolster us or send us reeling.

The doctors and nurses watched my sister for signs and symptoms of bleeding, especially tiny bloody splotches under her skin called petechiae, an indication of bleeding due to a low platelet count. Just as her platelet count was dropping, the same was true of her red blood cell count. As her blood count drifted lower, Victoria regularly received units of blood. The trigger to transfuse was a hemoglobin count that dropped below eight; a normal red blood count is in the range of twelve to fourteen. The nurses were vigilant about checking her vital signs, watching for symptoms of a low blood count (which could indicate anemia) such as tachycardia, an increased heart rate (above 100 at rest would be cause for concern), low blood pressure, or dizziness on standing. They also checked her temperature at regular intervals; with a low white blood count, she was at high risk for infections of any kind.

Every morning, an automated blood count was entered onto the whiteboard in Victoria's room, and later in the day on Monday, Wednesday, and Friday, a differential was also registered. This was a hand count of the types of white cells circulating in the blood. Her overall blood count was very low at 100 or 200, with normal being 4,000 to 10,000. From this, the pathologist would calculate the ANC, or absolute neutrophil count, which would generally run from 200 to 500, as well as the percentage of circulating blasts in her blood.

The ANC is a measure of the white cells available to fight bacterial infections. This number would determine whether Victoria could have visitors or, better yet, whether she could leave her hospital room. Anyone with illness was barred from visiting, as even a simple cold could kill her. With no ability to fight infection, she was at risk of fungal infections or sepsis caused by accidental cuts. During her stay in the hospital, and later, following her transplant, my sister was not allowed to eat any fresh food, especially things like salads and fruit, which she craved, because of the potential exposure to bacteria she would be unable to fight off.

The blast percent is a number indicating whether or not the chemotherapy is effective. When she was first diagnosed, Victoria's white count was over 30,000, with 40 percent blasts. As the chemotherapy killed off her white cells, the percentage of blasts decreased. Often this number would hover around 10 percent, but as the chemotherapy produced results, the blast percentage dropped to 2–3 percent and eventually to zero. Unlike the red cells and platelets, the white cells cannot be replaced. Drugs can stimulate white cell production, but giving these to patients with leukemia would stimulate the leukemia as well. It is not possible to transfuse someone else's white cells without causing a significant reaction of fever and illness.

Next on the board was a list of the active medications Victoria was receiving and a schedule for her day, which would include chemotherapy and infusions, as well as visits from physical therapists, spiritual counselors, social workers, and various other support staff. Before I'd arrived, Victoria had a peripherally inserted central catheter (PICC) line inserted into a vein in her right arm, extending to the superior vena cava, the large central vein returning blood to her heart. A Christmas tree of intravenous lines was connected to the PICC line, delivering steady infusions as well as "piggybacks," or dosages of drugs, which are attached to the infusion line. In addition, the PICC sent "pushes," drugs given throughout the course of the day, into the intravenous line. My sister was on three antibiotics, an antifungal infusion, and antiviral medications, in addition to her chemotherapy drugs.

The intravenous line assembly was her albatross; she had to tow it with her to the bathroom, and it stood sentry next to her bed while she slept. With a line assembly, things we take for granted, like changing clothes and showering, suddenly become complicated and require nursing assistance to disconnect and then reconnect the PICC line. All my sister's personal care was now scheduled by the hospital staff. Much of her day was occupied with the managing of her intravenous lines and pumps, calling for her nurse when an alarm would sound, waiting for the unit clerk to respond, and reporting the problem to the clerk, who would find the nurse, who would come to her room to correct the problem.

This seemed like a poorly choreographed dance that managed to inconvenience all parties. The time between crises could be five minutes or, with a little luck, several hours. Between the interruptions of the nurses, staff, dietary services, housekeeping, and ancillary personnel, it was difficult to get sustained rest. The interruptions went on throughout the day and night. This too, I realized, was part of life in the hospital. I was used to being up much of the night on call, but I always knew I would eventually leave and find my own pillow at home.

Chemotherapy can cause severe nausea and vomiting, depending on the agents being used to treat the cancer. Fortunately for Victoria, although she often had a low-grade nausea, she rarely vomited and generally was tolerating the medications quite well. When she spiked a fever, she would undergo a "fever workup," which included a battery of tests such as blood and urine cultures, nasal swabs, and chest X-rays. The thinking was to jump on any infection quickly, before it spun out of control. Rapid interventions could be made, either adding new antibiotics or changing the medications she was receiving. Fortunately, these fever workups were almost always negative.

Apart from enduring boredom, Victoria wanted reassurance that she would get better, that she would survive. She also wanted information and explanations about the drugs and treatments and their protocols. She wanted to know what was coming so that she could pace herself as she fought her way back to health. Her initial focus was getting through the chemotherapy, finding a donor, and then having the transplant. Next, there was a required three-month stay at City of Hope, where she would remain indoors and largely isolated. At the end, if all her blood counts and symptoms appeared normal, she would be able to return to Santa Monica and attempt to pick up her life where she had left off.

She was just restarting an acting career after a prolonged hiatus to raise her two boys and run the household. Earlier in her career she had appeared in multiple television shows, including *Law and Order* and *Boston Common*, and in a variety of stage productions. She'd also

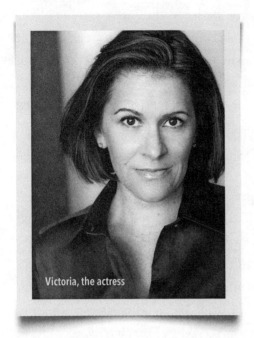

Victoria, the actress

starred in the award-winning short *Ladies' Room LA*, which she produced with Pat. Prior to her diagnosis she had begun auditioning again and was getting callbacks and being offered parts. Never the ingénue, she was an actor ahead of her years and had finally grown into the age of the characters she was most suited to play. Isolated at City of Hope, she wanted to get back to her family and the tremendous friendships she had cultivated. For Victoria, a profoundly social person, being cut off from her world and friends was a form of torture.

Victoria wanted to understand her disease in the abstract. What was AML, how did it work, how do white blood cells work, what are platelets, how do we produce blood products, where were the cancerous cells living in her body? She was impatient with her leukemia, since it had arrived uninvited from out of nowhere and taken over her life. She wanted to understand tumor suppressor genes and why she had developed leukemia in the first place. She wanted to understand what was happening, but also whether her illness could be passed to her children and what tests could be performed to protect them from a similar fate. Yet, while she wanted to learn more about AML as it related to heritability so that she might protect her children, at the same time she did not want to learn the specifics of the disease as it related to her.

I tiptoed around the elephant in my sister's stark white room, aware that she was stubbornly pushing away the idea of death. Victoria fully embraced her treatments, including her doctors and the goal of cure. She was at one of the best institutions available and statistics didn't matter—after all, she was not an actual statistic herself. Some people survived this illness, and she was going to be one of them.

She believed that attitude, focus, and complete commitment to cure would get her through and, ultimately, suffice. I worried that I would telegraph my skepticism, that she would read my face and see my fear and uncertainty, leaving her no choice but to acknowledge her dire predicament. Perhaps driven by her own terror, she did not seem to perceive my growing discomfort in the face of such dismal odds. I did not know how I would handle such a diagnosis myself.

In *When Blood Breaks Down: Life Lessons from Leukemia*, Mikkael Sekeres captures this attitude and the tension between hope and denial in patients diagnosed with leukemia: "People who choose to receive the most aggressive chemotherapy may choose to remember the best odds, or exaggerate those odds, to bolster the justification for their decision. Or, some may enter a type of adaptive denial to cope with both their diagnosis and the long-shot odds of chemotherapy curing them. A more positive spin on this coping mechanism is to call it optimism, or hope—both of which have been associated with better outcomes among cancer patients."

Hope is extremely important in surviving cancer. A good friend of mine, no stranger to adversity, who also trained as a neurosurgeon, once said, "There is no such thing as false hope; there is only hope." Victoria believed that she would recover. When we sat together in her room, she maintained her sense of humor, telling jokes and fondly recollecting events from our childhood. Our conversations meandered, moving freely between the present and our shared past. When the subject shifted back to her illness, I would answer her questions and stop when she no longer seemed interested or when she grew tired. I was grateful for my medical knowledge, even though I was not intimately versed in the treatments for leukemia. I felt I had something useful and concrete to offer.

At times, our chats about leukemia were no different from the interactions I have had with scores of patients and their families. I am often the first one to know that my patient has a malignant brain tumor. Laying out the truth and the treatment options with the family is part of my job, but it never gets easier. How do I tell the family while the patient is not present and is in the recovery room waking up from the immediate effects of anesthesia? Some families, as do patients, want to know everything, from prognosis to future treatments, while others want to know nothing at all. Hope and optimism are important drivers of survival and recovery. When patients ask, "How long do I have?" I am always reluctant to give a specific answer. The truth is, I don't know. And I may be wrong, either with the diagnosis or the prognosis.

Patients aren't statistics. They are individuals, and as such they are not bound by the accepted rules of an illness. Survival is always a range, and some people do recover from illnesses considered "fatal." I have long-term survivors of glioblastoma multiforme (GBM) in my practice, even though the majority of patients die within a year or two of diagnosis. Why some patients become outliers is often a mystery.

Knowledge and treatment options are continually changing and improving, so patients may get lucky. We may find a cure that will benefit them before they succumb to their disease. Yet the reality is that over the last twenty-five years, the improvement in survival for patients with high-grade gliomas and GBMs has been modest, without fundamental changes in the natural history of the disease.

We never want to extinguish hope, both for the patient and the practitioner. I want to believe that my patient will survive and be cured. I want to have hope as well, even when the survival data tell me otherwise. The survival data for AML with monosomy 7 carries a 6 percent five-year survival rate for all patients. Had Victoria known this, she would have focused on the six survivors, yet it is hard not to think of the ninety-four of the hundred who will die.

I spent the first weekend of the new year with my sister, catching up and reminiscing, and returned early Monday morning to meet Dr. O'Donnell. Anxious to hear more about Victoria's illness and the treatment program in store for her, which to date had been frustratingly nebulous, I felt that if I could meet the doctor in person, I might establish a rapport, perhaps trade email addresses. I needed my sister's blessing so that it would be clear to Dr. O'Donnell that my involvement was welcome and useful for her immediate family and also for our larger family, all of whom wanted information, felt starved for facts, and were hanging on every word.

Our brother-in-law, Gerald, sent me the link to a *New Yorker* article by Dr. Jerome Groopman describing exciting new developments in AML treatment. These treatments were leading to spectacular remissions and cures. Earlier on the phone, I had asked Dr. Fischer to test my sister's blood for IDH1 status—if the AML was IDH1-positive, this drug could be curative. I had already contacted the drug company; they were aware of my sister's leukemia and gave me relevant questions to ask. Apparently, City of Hope was registered to participate in a clinical trial of this drug but had yet to enroll their first patient.

When Dr. O'Donnell arrived in Victoria's room, she was wearing rubber gloves and a mask over her nose and mouth. Her speech was measured and careful, and her large brown eyes had a sad, knowing look. She was the opposite of the typical surgeon—often in a hurry, exuding confidence, whisking into the room already thinking about the next task. Dr. O'Donnell was polite and considerate and examined my sister carefully, deliberate and unhurried in her actions. She answered Victoria's questions, yet did not volunteer her own concerns. She was forthright, kind, and eminently practical. She seemed to be the perfect choice for my sister. I sensed this doctor genuinely appreciated Victoria's compliance with treatments and willingness to follow her recommendations.

After they finished, I followed the doctor into the hall and closed the door behind me. I expressed my concerns about the lack of communication and explained that I wished to interpret the facts of Victoria's leukemia to our family. She and I exchanged email addresses. The bone marrow results would be back soon, she said. These would include information about me and Caroline, along with the database of possible donors. Dr. O'Donnell agreed to check on the IDH1 status testing and said she would let me know the result. She acknowledged how difficult Victoria's leukemia was to treat and cure, but told me that with transplantation, my sister had up to a 40 percent chance of survival, which was much better than the 6 percent I had previously believed to be the case. Not great odds, but a lot better than I had thought.

The next day, Dr. O'Donnell returned to Victoria's room and informed us that neither Caroline nor I would be a suitable match for our sister. She also explained that Victoria's IDH1 status was negative, so the new trial drug was not an option. On her rounds the following morning, she broke the results of the database search. The provisional results indicated that of the twenty-two million potential donors tested, there was only one possible match. She apologized for the disappointing news, saying that they would keep searching for potential matches and might have some other possibilities, so we should not give up hope. While neither Caroline nor I would be suitable donors for Victoria, in a strange twist of fate, the tests showed that we were both matches for each other. Caroline was devastated by this news, having wished that she could become Victoria's donor and save her life. I was stunned and scared, knowing that the search for a donor in the wider world would prove to be a game of long odds.

I have now been here for one and a half weeks. I've done my second round of chemo and a repeat bone marrow biopsy (my third), and next Wednesday we see if I am in remission or not. My first biopsy showed that my marrow was so caked with disease that it couldn't even aspirate.

The second was far easier, but the blast numbers were still very present.

Now I am praying for zero—for remission. If that is my good luck, I will get to go home for one to two weeks before another three to five weeks for the apparently grueling transplant.

Yesterday morning, Dr. O'Donnell came in and remarked, first thing, "Your siblings match each other but not you." What a cruel pronouncement. Crazy cruel. Dr. O said that when she started doing this, if you didn't have a sibling match, you were out of luck. Good thing it is 2015, so there are other options. Now I am praying for (1) remission so I can go home and regroup for a short time and (2) a match! A perfect, excellent match with a healthy p53 gene!

So there we have it.

Valerie [a close friend] wrote me a lovely prayer. She said my trials and tribulations "now amount to a cliffhanger," which inspired her to write the following:

> *I ask for a most benevolent outcome that the perfect and ideal donor for my bone marrow transplant be found speedily and may the results of the procedure be better and easier and more powerfully healing than I could hope for or expect.*

Love that! I'd also like to add that I get one to two weeks off in between so I can recapture my spirit (being with my men) and my energy (being out of the hospital!) first. If I am not in remission, I'll have to go straight into more chemo and/or radiation—which is concerning in terms of energy and also secondary cancers . . .

I really don't want to be a watched pot, forever worrying about my body. I say no more cancer, ever. I like what Nick said, "The third time is the charm, Mom."   —JANUARY 1, 2015

There is a lot of hurry up and wait in this dance. Dr. O'Donnell came this morning with no news. Apparently, the matching folks were not working yesterday or on the first. No surprise; it is not the best time of the year to be sick! Now we may need to wait until Monday for any news of a match . . .

I'm doing okay right now. I woke up feeling awful, but now I'm feeling well enough. I woke up thinking I was going to throw up again and feeling very congested. Now, I am better, except that I am bored and going ever so slightly out of my mind. As I remarked to Pat, "Why can't people be in an induced coma for the wiping out of the bone marrow part?" Although I have heard that it can be the posttransplant part that can actually be the most challenging—the period that brings challenges with graft vs. host disease. I guess my rash could be seen as a preview of things to come.

I am just really hoping that:

- I'm in remission—can go home and snuggle with my boys for a bit and avoid more chemo and radiation, which is not great for "secondary cancers," plus will make me weak.
- We find a great match ASAP. No more of this torturous waiting!

I am grateful for:

- The kind nurses caring for me.
- My amazing, loving, and supportive husband who just went off to Target to try to find me sleep bras! (That's much worse than asking him to buy tampons at CVS.)
- My incredibly brave and strong boys.
- The kindness of family who flew in to help—Deanna, Joe, my mom, Caroline, Gerald, Cass, and now Jody, with many more standing by.
- And friends—so many have been completely amazing. Alison, Diane, Jen, Heather, Mira, Lisa D., Cat Gerst, Laura and Scott, Trish, Jenny, Holli—so, so many!

—JANUARY 2, 2015

Victoria had entered a maze with too many dead ends. Paths to a cure were gradually being closed off, choices becoming limited. While I was inspired by my sister's optimism, I knew that it would not be enough to counter the losses she was facing. As much as I tried, I could not push away my increasing sense of dread.

During my second visit to City of Hope (shortly after her transplant), a North Carolina neighbor who serves on the hospital board arranged a tour for me of the research facilities and the adjoining hospitals. I was enormously appreciative of the opportunity. Patients come from all over the country for the best possible treatments; staff often drive hours to and from the hospital to care for their patients. The physicians and researchers have an almost religious conviction to their mission and vision.

What I had initially perceived as coldness from some of the physicians I began to recognize as self-preservation. I suspect Dr. O'Donnell knew that my sister was likely to die before she had even met her. Despite this, she was invested in Victoria's care, bringing her experience and expertise to bear. How hard would it be to grow attached to patients and their families, only to lose so many of them in death? Even with the most heroic efforts and state-of-the-art medical treatments, many patients succumb to their illnesses and die. The chance of a breakthrough and the desire to ease suffering propels doctors like O'Donnell. For the treating physician, there is always another patient who needs help, another family with questions, another experiment to run with the possibility of a cure.

During Victoria's stay, City of Hope staged a reunion of leukemia and bone marrow transplant survivors, filling the garden patio with grateful former patients and their families. My sister watched from her window, inspired by what she saw playing out beneath her, a thin pane of glass separating her from the freedom from disease she craved.

The question with no good answer hangs in the air: why did they make it while I might not? How many want to ask: why did I get leukemia in the first place? Most of those patients and their families had no familiarity with leukemia upon the diagnosis and found themselves thrust into a world of medical chemistry they had no desire to enter. One of the greatest things that came of the City of Hope reunion was the connections the patients made with one another, as well as with their own families. The renewed relationship I had with my sister was uplifting and full of meaning. With cancer, priorities shift suddenly and small gifts of time together become more important than anything money can buy.

Caroline and I had desperately hoped to be matches for Victoria. The fact that she would not be the donor was a blow for Caroline, as mentioned, but it crushed Victoria as well. One of the hardest things about mortal illness in a family member is the helplessness one feels as everything unfolds. It's like watching a slow-motion car crash: your impulse is to jump in and do something, yet you find yourself incapable of changing the hands of fate. Much as we want to intervene, we feel powerless against the seeming inevitability of a disease's progression.

My ability to explain things to my family allowed me to feel useful. Caroline now felt that she had nothing to offer Victoria, so the idea that her cells could save our younger sister's life had been deeply important to her. The loss of that hope felt like a great personal failing. When we were informed that Caroline and I were matches for each other but neither was a match for Victoria, insult was added to helplessness.

On finding that she was not a donor, Caroline went to work contacting charitable Jewish bone marrow donation organizations, including Gift of Life, which exists to match patients in need with registered donors. She was all set to run bone marrow drives through her synagogue, and plans were rapidly developed to run drives at the boys' school in Los Angeles as well.

These plans never took off because, despite the willingness of all participants, it became clear that the odds of finding a donor this way were infinitesimal. Also—and this became the biggest factor—the timing wouldn't work. Dr. O'Donnell explained that by the time we organized a drive, got the samples, and had them evaluated, Victoria would likely be beyond the window for transplantation. The longer she waited, the more likely it was that her leukemia would progress or that she would develop superinfections due to a prolonged state of impaired immunity. If she developed even one of these infections, transplantation would be eliminated as an option altogether.

Nonetheless, a call went out to our extended family and to our half-sisters, Madeleine and Alex, who immediately volunteered to be tested. Both sisters turned out to be matches for Victoria. Initially, the doctors at City of Hope were leaning more toward Madeleine than Alex, but all communication about possible donors was painfully slow and we would often wait several weeks for answers to our questions.

To our surprise, in late February, Dr. O'Donnell asked for Victoria and Pat's son Nick to be tested. He was fifteen at the time.

Nick is the older of Victoria and Pat's two sons. He is quiet, sensitive, and extremely kind. He was acutely aware of the seriousness of his mother's situation. Both boys were trying to adapt to her long absences. Pat and Victoria struggled to keep their home as normal as possible during her illness, but as treatment and hospitalizations dragged on, this became a tremendous challenge. Pat divided his time between home and hospital while his work and health suffered. Without the generosity of friends and neighbors, these months would have been close to impossible, but the boys also met the challenge, becoming more self-sufficient and considerate. Nick stepped up his role as a big brother to Will, and together they helped their dad keep the household running.

Both Pat and Victoria were initially worried when Nick was mentioned as a possible donor. As a fifteen-year-old, would he be emotionally able to handle this? Would he be devastated if he were found not to be a match? What if he was a match and the transplant went forward and failed? Would he forever carry a burden of guilt and a sense of responsibility? What if Nick was injured in the process of harvesting his bone marrow? It is hard for a parent to expose a child to pain and risk for the parent's benefit.

While Nick would not be a complete match, recent data have shown that haplotypes (half-matches) can be effective donors. Plus, there is a developing appreciation that young males often make the best donors since they produce large volumes of healthy stem cells. In the past, donors were put under general anesthesia and then had up to forty bone marrow biopsies taken from their pelvis. There were risks of bleeding, fracture, nerve injury, and complications related to the anesthesia. The procedure was notoriously painful. Today, donors receive daily injections of Filgrastim, a drug that stimulates the production of white blood cells, for a week, followed by up to six hours of plasmapheresis, in which the donor's blood is circulated through a filtration system that captures circulating stem cells. These are concentrated, saved, and then infused into the recipient after their own marrow has been destroyed with powerful chemotherapy and high-dose radiation.

Dr. O'Donnell pointed out that most people end up with a few possible matches, but a few unlucky patients end up with none. We waited for over two weeks for news about the lone potential donor. It later became clear that the potential donor was not interested in participating. Since this is all done with complete anonymity, we were not able to contact or learn anything about her or him. We did not know the person's age, sex, location, or any other identifying features.

Almost ten weeks in the hospital. Twelve weeks since I went to the ER with, perhaps, the flu! That is a lot of time alone. It is wearing on me more now. Perhaps because it has been so terribly long, perhaps because the transplant is drawing nearer (I think!). I am definitely struggling more. It is a jumble of so many things.

So much time away from my family. It is getting harder to turn it around and see the beauty around me and feel the gratitude. Right now, I feel incredulous, still astonished that this ever happened, distinctly aware of how many blows there have been. One of my friends said I was going to suffer from posttraumatic stress disorder when this was all over since it started with such a bang and there has been so little opportunity to process it all.

How is it possible that Caroline and Jody match each other and not me? How is it possible in a database of twenty-four million that there was only one potential donor match? And how is it possible that this one potential donor is not available for further testing when I need him or her?

I will just have to trust my doctors. If they choose haplo and I have graft-versus-host issues, that will be what is needed. If I have to take handfuls of immunosuppressing drugs all of my life, so be it. I will be here and that is all that matters. I will do whatever it takes. I am determined to be here until I have reached a ripe old age. I have so much left to do. I have roles to play, books to write, projects to produce, but most of all, people to love and nurture.

I am nowhere close to done. Not an option. Wow, what a mosaic of fear, shock, loss, strength, confidence, love, and gratitude I am right now. A smorgasbord of emotions, many of them a lot less positive than usual. But as my acting teacher Rudi Shelly used to say: "Even Plato had occasionally to go to the loo." I've felt amazingly positive and strong. I still do. But other feelings are definitely creeping in.   —FEBRUARY 21, 2015

Can I just say the food delivery people drive me crazy? The forced chipperness is super-annoying. I like one of the women—she just comes in quietly, says good morning, and sets down my tray. I so appreciate her. The hairnet dude this morning just entered with a "Good morning! Well, you're up bright and early this morning!" Really? It's a hospital, dude. It's 7:30 a.m.! Most of us are up at 4 or 5. I know he means well, but please, leave me alone! Of course it is far worse at the City of Hope when they enter, announcing, "Room service!" They check my name and date of birth as if I was going to sneak into someone else's bed and eat their food? Oy.

Today, I was feeling fearful, and [Sherry, the chaplain] helped walk me back to my place of peace. She said that fear is (1) thoughts and (2) listening to the thoughts, which lead to (3) fear. She said the antidote is to step aside (I am rephrasing) and go back inside—that inside is the garden that needs to be cultivated, seeds planted, and that therein lies the peace.

I am mad at Hitler all over again. I think the notes must be somewhere else, on a scrap of paper? I know I took notes after meeting with the rabbi, Janet, at Sherry's suggestion. The discussions began in conversation with Diane about the shockingly low number, a mere thirteen million, of Jews in the world. Many of those are Sephardic. Fewer are Ashkenazi. How, if Hitler had not wiped out six million, there would be so many more Jews in the world now. To my astonishment, there is no match for me in the database of twenty-four million.   —FEBRUARY 24, 2015

I am feeling so scared these days. Scared for the transplant and scared about after. I am scared that my p53 gene is mutated, and scared that I will be getting total body radiation. I am terrified of getting another problem after I resolve this one. So utterly and completely unfair.

Jody said I need the radiation, no discussion. He had also said way back in the beginning that if I didn't do what they told me and tried some Eastern approach, as is so much more my orientation, he would come to Santa Monica and drag me there himself.   —MARCH 4, 2015

I had to return to North Carolina before any of the details of transplantation had been worked out. It would end up taking until early March before a final decision about the transplant donor had been made. They eliminated the MUD (matched unrelated donor) for reasons we did not fully understand and were considering Madeleine's or Nick's cells, or cord blood samples that had been found to be a good potential match. Cord blood refers to banked umbilical cord blood from unrelated newborns (unless the mother has chosen to bank cord blood at the time of birth, which Victoria had not done). Cord blood is full of stem cells, which can be amplified and have been shown to be an effective option in the absence of matched donors.

In the end, Dr. O'Donnell announced that the transplant committee at City of Hope had decided on Nick as the donor and they wanted to prepare him for donation at the end of March. The pretransplant conditioning for Victoria would take place at the same time, with transplantation scheduled in early April. This latest turn was jarring, since Nick was not an exact match and he was significantly younger than most donors.

Victoria had completed one round of chemotherapy, followed by a predictable bottoming out of her blood counts. Dr. O'Donnell waited for these to rebound so that Victoria could undergo a bone marrow biopsy to determine the effectiveness of the chemotherapy drugs. If there was no evidence of leukemic cells in her biopsy, then it would be possible for her to return home for a week or two before readmission to the hospital for a second round of conditioning chemotherapy. Once she made it through this course, she would be ready for the transplant. I was advised to return a week or two after the transplant, since this would be the most precarious time for my sister. With Pat's blessing this time, I booked my flights. I was relieved to know that I could be of use.

The bone marrow results were provisionally encouraging, with abundant monocytes and next to no blasts. They let Victoria go home for almost two weeks before she was readmitted to Dr. Fischer's service at Saint John's for another round of chemotherapy. This would be far less disruptive than readmitting her all the way across LA. Genetic testing had to be performed on the bone marrow sample, so Victoria was called back to City of Hope for another biopsy to determine whether the few blasts that were present were immature normal white blood cells, which start out life as blasts, or leukemic cells with a deletion of chromosome 7, which would indicate that the chemotherapy had not worked at all.

The results suggested the leukemia was in check, so Victoria was allowed to take her next chemotherapy at Saint John's prior to being discharged home. If all went well, she would at last be released home to rest before her transplant. She sent me a celebratory text in all caps pointing out that this was the first time she had been able to leave the hospital in ten weeks.

transplant/ second visit

Poor, sweet Nick, I am so very sorry to have to drag you into this. Poor is the wrong word though—I know he will be fine, but I do regret having to involve him. He can do this—both emotionally and physically. Kathryn was so funny and so right when she said Nick would have a great essay for his college apps. And her comment was made before he became the Donor!

I had two burning questions for Dr. O: Nick and radiation. I will feel so much better if I can get the targeted radiation—targeting my bone marrow, not my entire body.

I have done CT studies, X-rays, heart studies, and a pulmonary study where I had to blow into a plastic tube, hold my breath, etc., to measure my lung function. Pat and I attended a class describing what to expect during the BMT [bone marrow transplant]. We had a consult with Meredith, the social worker who works with Dr. O. . . . I very much appreciate Meredith's no-nonsense approach, and I like her very much . . .

I told her I could hear some of the stuff I should watch out for but said that I didn't want to hear about death. We spoke, briefly, about how you can sometimes spend time in the ICU during your transplant, you can get rehospitalized during the hundred days, that you always puke . . . And then, at the very end, she just had to throw in a "sometimes people pass away . . ." I should have called her on it. Perhaps it is a liability thing where you need to be informed?

And she mentioned risk of relapse and recurrence. Okay, that is not an option. One year, two and a half years, and five years are important milestones. If you get to two and a half years, apparently you only have a 5 percent chance of recurrence.

I am having yet another bone marrow biopsy this Friday. I am definitely anxious about that. I feel fine. There is no reason to worry, but it does have my attention. Of course, my bone marrow is often twitching,

but I have learned that happens when it comes back to life—throughout
this process.   —MARCH 18, 2015

I am still in stunned shock after yesterday. So much. I saw a glimmer of just
how beat up I am going to be. First of all, we had Nick in tow, so Pat really
had to focus on him. This is intense stuff with which he has to deal. Pat said
that all day long people were telling Nick what a hero he is. The people
helping and testing him went out of their way to treat him really well.

My day began with my fourth bone marrow biopsy—or was it my
fifth? My low back is super-unhappy this morning. Dr. O came to visit me
in recovery. She said they will let me do the targeted radiation. It turns
out she had to lobby for this and the head of the radiology department
had to approve. They have been doing targeted radiation for ten years,
and I believe the head of radiology created the method, but they have
never used it on someone in my particular situation. I believe it has been
used previously with sicker patients, people in much worse shape than I. I
believe more people will do this in the future. This all came about because
Jody had read about this and thought it was better for me . . .

. . . I pushed for it, and then all of a sudden there I was, being
measured for it—and it is horrible. They created a mold for my legs to
hold them in place, and fitted a mask to my face that gets screwed into
place, bolting me to the table. The mask fits so snugly that I now have
bright red dots—bruises—on my chin. These are from the circles in the
mask through which I will be able to breathe.

I look like I'm wearing Klingon makeup from a Star Trek episode!
And they tattooed my skin in seven places! When one of the staff said he
was going to tattoo me, I thought he was joking; he wasn't. All of this is to
secure me into position so I will always be in this exact same configuration
so that the radiation rays will always hit the exact same marks. It took one
and a half hours to fit me. It was freaky and awful.

I pushed to make this happen, so now I've just got to trust that it
makes more sense. Although some elements might be tougher up front, I
am hoping that it will be far better for my body in the long run.

As for my dear, sweet son, I was very proud of him. I said to Nick that
it is kind of his choice how hard or not hard this is—that's really the point of
this book [Victoria's goal for her journal was to see it published], that there
is a valuable life lesson in mastering this concept [of how hard things must
be]. I said to him that it is true in tennis as well—that he can continue to
complain about Jeremiah, his doubles partner, or he can trust that they are
improving and growing together as a team and that they will improve over
time. The first day we took Nick to City of Hope for testing, we had to stop

the car for an emergency bathroom break, as he had gotten himself in quite a state. He was infinitely calmer on our drive back yesterday morning.

They took twelve vials of his blood, poked and prodded him a lot, and he handled it fine. I feel like he really took my advice to heart. It was so much easier on him! —MARCH 21, 2015

I do think there is something larger at work here—something to do with a life calling / a role I will play. Not only do I need to stick around for my family, but also I have much still to offer. Today, saying goodbye to the boys as they set off . . . with their five cousins and one amazing Aunt Barb, I was less emotional than anticipated. They were crying and hugging me tightly—whereas I was memorizing their feel, their touch, their sweet breath against my cheek, their salty tears. I was memorizing every bit of them in case I ever need to recall these sensations as a reminder of what, precisely, I intend to stick around for. They need me; Pat does, too. And I need them. —MARCH 28, 2015

Dr. O'Donnell said the slides came back from the bone marrow biopsy and they detected 1 percent of the "bad actor" 7 chromosomes—the monosomy 7. They are supposed to be in pairs, and in some I am missing one half of the pair.

My head is reeling with this new info. Would this have happened if I'd gone to transplant faster? Or was it just in hiding before? And how does this impact things? Scary. I'm so sad and mad. And yet, is it a surprise? I have been told and have known that the monosomy 7 chromosomal abnormality is of a trickier variety with a higher chance of recurrence, so isn't this just showing me how that is the case? This is certainly showing me how necessary is the transplant.

And there is no reason not to assume that the transplant won't eradicate every last "bad actor" cell. The preparation should get rid of the bad cells, as it will wipe out my bone marrow entirely. And the new bone marrow should fight off any errant cell. Right?

I had some chocolate just now, but that didn't really help. I thought about scotch, but I refrained. I'm very disciplined. —MARCH 30, 2015

After three months, everything was set for Victoria's transplant. Nick rose to the occasion, and Joe and Deanna, his uncle and aunt, gave him daily shots to stimulate production of stem cells. Just as Victoria had developed aches and a fever with the onset of her leukemia, Nick developed bone pain, but other than missing a few days of school he managed without any untoward complications.

Most doctors, including hematologists and oncologists, have limited exposure to bone marrow transplantation; this is considered a highly specialized, technical, pioneering area of medicine. Dr. Fischer answered candidly that he was out of his depth when I asked him specific questions about my sister's impending transplant. There are a few areas of medicine that tend to provoke fear in most doctors. Neurosurgery is one; burn medicine is another; and transplant, in particular bone marrow transplant, is a third. This is generally a quaternary service where even large health systems refer patients to specialized centers. While I am comfortable in the world of neurosurgery, I share a comparable fear of bone marrow transplantation and burn medicine.

Victoria was admitted to City of Hope's transplant unit on March 31. She was given three rounds of high-dose chemotherapy to kill off her bone marrow, which caused nausea and tremendous fatigue. Palifermin, a drug to protect her mucosal surfaces, was administered because the chemotherapy and radiation could make her slough off her mucosal lining (mouth and intestinal tract) and develop ulcers. Radiation to her entire skeleton would follow with TomoTherapy. TomoTherapy is a CT-driven high-dose radiation therapy that would target her skeleton and spare her solid organs, such as her brain, heart, and intestines.

(*Victoria:* On April 9, 2015, a day before the transplant, the day of Nick's apheresis, I must have written him this note.)

My Darling Nick,
Thank you so much for what you are doing for me. It is a phenomenal gift. You are brave and strong and I couldn't be more proud of you. What a strong and loving son! I couldn't ask for anything more.
I love you forever,
Mom

On the back was his reply:

Hey, Mom,
This isn't so bad. It's totally worth it. ILU so much.
   Nick
   PS: Sorry about my handwriting . . . writing is harder! ILU!

(Writing was harder since he'd been hooked up to machines all day.)

The transplant took place on April 10, after a brutal week of preparation. They had hoped to extract 5 million cells from Nick, but he produced 16.2 million. The stem cells looked like a milky suspension of cloudy blood in an IV bag. Over a few hours the new cells were sent through Victoria's PICC line, slowly incorporating into her system. She was given a new birthday of April 10.

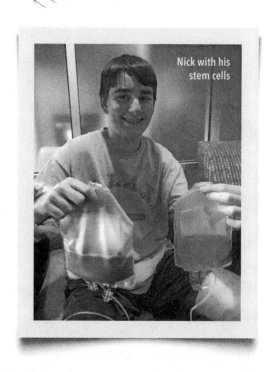

Nick with his stem cells

TRANSPLANT DAY

Today is my new birthday. It is here. I began my day feeling dreadful after the fourth night of fever and chills. I had a CT scan, which confirmed fluid in my lungs. I am now taking two new antibiotics. My fever last night was 102.5°. My bedding and clothing were drenched and required multiple changings.

Pat put his head on my chest and played "Ooh Child," by the Five Stairsteps, and wept. We cried together.

I'm feeling better than earlier now. We are waiting for "the bag," which feels a tad anticlimactic.

They needed 5 million stem cells from Nick, would have settled with 4 million, but he produced 16.2 million! Dr. O said that is enough for three

81

people! They are going to freeze half of his cells in case I should ever need more down the road. (No, thank you—won't be needed.) Nick's unfrozen cells are en route as we speak.   —APRIL 10, 2015

She continued to spike fevers each night, along with drenching sweats, shivering chills, and rigors. She developed a rash on her chest, possibly due to fevers or a side effect of the radiation treatments. She was restarted on multiple intravenous antibiotics along with antirejection drugs around the clock. She was not, by any means, out of the woods.

I arrived during the third week of April to relieve Pat and sit by my sister's bedside. I was more apprehensive than I had been in January because I didn't know what to expect. In the hallway I scrubbed my hands, gowned, and gloved, and then entered her room. Victoria was confined to her bed. All color had drained from her face. She was impossibly pale. Though she was battling continuous nausea and aching throughout her body, she tried to muster up some enthusiasm for my visit, but it was clearly an effort. She had no appetite because food only made her nausea worse. Simple things like making it to the bathroom required focused energy, as if she were climbing a mountain at high altitude. She was easily winded, profoundly weak.

Her high fevers persisted, so Dr. O'Donnell ordered a chest CT scan that showed a fluid collection in her lungs. Her team was concerned about the possibility of a fungal infection in her chest, so the next day she underwent a bronchoscopy. While Victoria was sedated, a pulmonologist inserted a fine tube into her lung and took tissue samples and washings to assess for signs of infection. They didn't find any signs of serious infection. Surprisingly, after that procedure her fever broke. She continued with labored breathing and required frequent inhalers, but no supplemental oxygen. Gradually, the shortness of breath abated and her breathing began to return to normal. This coincided with the addition of a second antifungal drug to her IV cocktail of medications.

Each day her white blood count climbed, which is a sign of engraftment, implying that the transplant was starting to take. By April 26, the count had returned to 2.0 from barely detectable. Presumably her leukemia was gone, so they had started Filgrastim to encourage white cell production. However, on April 29, she developed fevers up to 102.5° again and received a transfusion of red cells and platelets. She experienced chest pressure and was started on supplemental oxygen. They administered steroids for her pain, as well as diuretics for all the intravenous fluids she was receiving so she would be able to get rid of the excess, which was causing puffiness in her legs and bloating.

Watching someone undergoing treatment for leukemia after a bone marrow transplant is like watching a cooking show from hell. Sometimes in the hospital, particularly in the ER, I felt like a short-order cook, but this was ridiculous. Victoria had a seemingly unlimited number of intravenous infusions, including three antibiotics; two antifungal drugs; two antiviral medications; drugs to prevent rejection; steroids;

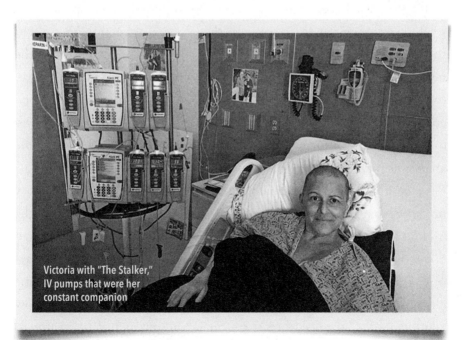

Victoria with "The Stalker," IV pumps that were her constant companion

and diuretics—not to mention blood products of platelets and red cells, and drugs like Filgrastim. She spent most of her time in bed, mired in a listless state of quasi-awareness and pain. Despite all of this, her spirits remained strong and upbeat. To my astonishment, she was never short-tempered or self-pitying. She was cooperative and polite to the nurses and aides, despite frequent interruptions at all times of the day and night. I was proud of the way my sister was handling herself, knowing the enormous stress and uncertainty she was facing. She remained determined to beat leukemia and girded herself for everything that was being thrown at her.

Victoria was enormously grateful to her caregivers and family and friends. Every day since she had entered the hospital, one of a large circle of friends dropped meals off at the Whelan home back in Santa Monica. They placed a cooler on the front porch that was invariably overflowing with healthy, delicious dinners, each carefully labeled to accommodate Will's allergies. Pat's family was especially supportive and spent many weeks camped out at their house so that Pat could be with Victoria at the hospital. He was juggling the responsibilities of his business, the needs of his sons, his wife's illness, and his own heart condition. I began to see, firsthand, the toll a prolonged illness takes on a family or even entire communities. The love and care my sister's family received was overwhelming. We made sure to count our blessings; many sick people are not as fortunate to have so many resources and devoted friends.

One afternoon, Victoria and I watched the third part of a documentary on cancer that had aired on PBS the previous month, based on Siddhartha Mukherjee's 2011 book, *The Emperor of All Maladies: A Biography of Cancer*. Some of the earlier episodes were depressing, covering the darker days of cancer treatments that ranged from radical surgery to devastating chemotherapies. They showed the ineffectiveness of bone marrow transplants for advanced breast cancer in the recent past, a treatment strategy now abandoned. This third installment looked to the future, toward potential areas of enormous promise, such as immunotherapy and, more specifically, less toxic therapies for cancer.

The problem with Victoria's treatment, from chemotherapies to transplant, was a dearth of knowledge. We currently do not know enough to conquer this disease with any elegance. So much of what we do in cancer treatment is nonselective and unrefined. The drugs we use attack the most rapidly dividing cells in the body, fundamentally damaging them by inserting mutations into their DNA. When this is done in the leukemic cells it is beneficial, yet when it occurs in otherwise normal cells it is harmful. Even if they undergo successful treatment and cure of their disease, leukemia patients are at risk for secondary malignancies that are the direct result of the curative treatments they have gone through, which damage both normal and abnormal DNA.

Immunotherapy is a way to master signaling within the body so that a cancer cell will elicit a response that causes or encourages the body's own defenses to take over and kill the abnormal cell. Because cancer cells are "us," the body often lacks the ability to recognize them as a threat. Immunotherapy offers the promise of triggering such a response within the patient. If only we'd had the tools to undo the mutation that led to Victoria's leukemia, or to mark these mutant cells as foreign and dangerous so that the body could use its internal defenses to rid itself of these abnormal cells, she might not have required a transplant in the first place. Despite great advances in the treatment of leukemia, the treatments are still plagued with limitations and brutal side effects.

Victoria was receptive to the potential of a bright future in cancer care. She was focused on that horizon. When I spoke with her about the possibility that she might die from this illness, she immediately shut me down. This was simply not going to happen to her. I let it drop, but I was troubled by her unwillingness to consider death. This was one of her ground rules: I would answer her medical questions and interpret the journey she and her family found themselves on, but I could not suggest that she might not survive. It was a tacit agreement between us, and I didn't have the confidence to press her.

My sister continued to channel all of her energy into being the most compliant patient she could be, religiously following her doctors' instructions, doing absolutely everything she could in order to live. She repeated, almost as a mantra, that she needed to live for the sake of her husband and their sons. It seemed to me that Victoria felt it was a sign of weakness to explore the idea of dying. She had indicated to Dr. O'Donnell and Dr. Fischer that she was not willing to discuss the notion of her death. She was giving treatment her all, and she was going to win!

> I just called Pat in tears and he was, of course, sympathetic, but in ending, he told me to stay strong. It is interesting that the conversation can be entirely different depending on whom you call. My mom, for example, would have taken me down a path of how hard this all is. Pat always wants to fix things—in general terms, isn't that more male?
>
> I watched the third episode of *The Emperor of All Maladies* with Jody just now. He deemed the first two too depressing but the final one uplifting. It was certainly interesting, as they are doing so many innovative things with immunotherapy, among other things. Jody said something along the lines of how I am not in control of this. I beg to differ. I believe our minds are powerful allies and that we don't have to simply roll over and wait for things to play out as they will.   —APRIL 22, 2015

It seemed to me that my sister's refusal to admit the possibility of defeat denied her family a chance to plan and to say goodbye. I'm not sure this would have softened their loss, but I like to think it would have helped mitigate some of the shock and despair that came with her sudden death. People who are willing to consider their own mortality seem more prepared and accepting of their fates.

As a society, we often interpret death as failure, yet we will all die of something. Have we perhaps overmedicalized the concepts of life and death, so that death has come to represent a treatment failure? Accepting death as natural and unavoidable both enriches our lives and allows us to make balanced decisions about when to treat diseases and when to change course toward palliation and comfort. Often, as was the case for Victoria, the treatments have toxicities and detrimental side effects. If they cease to work or if the potential damage outweighs the potential benefits, we need to consider whether to continue with treatments. If we regard progression of disease as an inherent failure, we will tend toward pushing treatment rather than pausing to have those difficult discussions about discontinuing therapies with limited benefit. This avoidance applies both to patients and their doctors.

As with many things in medicine, short-term suffering is required for the potential of long-term benefit. This pertains to surgeries as well as chemotherapies for cancer. Many of the side effects Victoria endured, which were actually the source of her symptoms, were the result of her treatments rather than the leukemia itself. Her declining blood counts, fevers and chills, painful rashes, and burns were all the result of damage inflicted on her normal systems in an effort to kill the leukemic cells. She hit her nadir when there were few, if any, circulating leukemic cells in her blood, but it was the specter of their return that motivated her and her doctors to push forward.

My numbers have begun to rise! WBC [white blood cell count] is 0.5! Yahoo. I am so encouraged.

I seldom watch *Grey's Anatomy* and stumbled upon it Thursday night. I was quite surprised that Dr. McDreamy was killed off. I thought of it just now and began to cry. I don't think it is really about Derek. I think it's the good news about my WBC.

I also think the tears are a lot about how moved I am that Jody spent so much time at my side. He has become a truly kind man with whom I feel very close. I felt like I got my brother back. He wasn't gone before, but we were both caught up in our busy lives and we hadn't made seeing each other priority. I believe that has shifted now.

Jody wrote to me in a text: "Be strong, my sister. I will miss you, and I am sorry to be heading home. You are everything a brother could wish for." Wow. And then, "It has been my pleasure to spend time with you. It is I who should be thanking you for allowing me the opportunity to be with you. I agree that future visits should be in a more pleasant place. But I will tell you that City of Hope is a special place. You have wonderful people looking after you, and for the time being, it is exactly what you need." Later, "I am really pleased about your white blood count. That is really good news. You are going to beat this, Toria!"

A few other exchanges followed, mostly about how great, nice, and funny our boys are. "Talk to you soon. I'm proud of you and your toughness." And then later, "While extremely difficult, in a way, what you're going through is a gift. The clarity you have achieved is unusual, as is the sense of meaning. Most people go through life in a fog or confused about what really matters, distracted by baubles and trinkets. Spending these two weeks with you has been a delight for me. I have grown as well, and I thank you for that. I believe I will be able to bring some of these realizations to other areas of my life and that this will be helpful on many levels." —APRIL 25, 2015

CHAPTER SIX

leukemia returns:
in memoriam

We all know that something is eternal. And it ain't houses and it ain't
names, and it ain't earth, and it ain't even the stars. . . . Everybody knows in
their bones that something is eternal, and that something has to do with
human beings. All the greatest people ever lived have been telling us that
for five thousand years and yet you'd be surprised how people are always
losing hold of it. There's something way down deep that's eternal about
every human being.   —THORNTON WILDER, *OUR TOWN*

After her diagnosis, Victoria asked me to relay information to our
extended family because she tired rapidly and lacked the energy to
respond to frequent phone calls and emails. Pat would send out useful,
succinct emails updating the family as soon as there were any significant
developments. With the cytogenetic testing and the determination of
monosomy 7 as the underlying mutation came questions and anguish.

As a physician, I find these conversations extremely difficult. No
matter how many times I find myself sitting across from a patient
preparing to break bad news, I always wonder how best to navigate this
sad and pivotal moment. How much should I say? What do they really
want to know? How much and when do I involve the family members?
Addressing the understandable fear and shock in a forthright,
compassionate way has taken years of practice. This is particularly
difficult when the patient is a child; I find the tone and the depth of

the conversation depends on the young person's age and maturity. I have to make a lot of quick assessments about how much information to volunteer, especially in the early stages of an unfavorable diagnosis. I take into account the extent of education and medical training that families bring to the conversation and try to present the facts and options as clearly as possible. Medical personnel speak a common language; they understand the data patterns and generally have a good sense of what the diagnosis of a specific illness implies.

When presenting bad information, I am always hesitant to speak about the patient without involving him or her in the discussion. But many patients specifically ask me to discuss their situations with their families and leave them out. My sister was insistent on limiting her awareness of survival rates and all the ways her treatment could potentially fail. Other patients feel the need to defer to their religious beliefs under these circumstances, adding a deeply personal and spiritual element to their choices about care.

As the weeks turned into months, my sister would ask me to discuss her blood counts with Pat, but not with her. She worried about the implications of bad news, as there was a tendency to hang on to every result. The blood counts and blast percentage would often set the tone for the day. She decided early on that she didn't find this information useful and figured that if she needed blood, they would give it to her. If not, they wouldn't. So often, patients and their families obsess over every data point they see, imbuing lab results with greater significance than they deserve. In the world of treatment, patients and their families often feel they have fallen down a rabbit hole.

This attention to numbers is particularly true in the ICU with telemetry, where respiratory rate, pulse, and blood pressure measurements (i.e., the vital signs) are prominently displayed in real time but often have little meaning in the larger picture. Our vital signs change a great deal during the day, with heart rates dropping into the high thirties when a fit person is sleeping. Similarly, heart rates will shoot up when a person is excited, upset, or in pain. The trends are usually what matters, rather than the momentary observations and minutiae.

Our mother took Victoria's diagnosis very hard. They had supported each other through the death of my mother's second husband, Jack, as well as through Pat's multiple open-heart surgeries. They spoke on the phone often. Approaching eighty, she had just lost both of her sisters and a close "double" cousin. A dear friend and walking partner had recently died of dementia. My mother appeared frail. I was worried about how she would handle the stress of Victoria's illness. I was hesitant to tell her everything I knew, but she was adamant about my not withholding information, no matter how bleak it might be. She wept into the telephone when I explained the prognosis of Victoria's type of leukemia. My father, while shaken, dutifully waited for the group updates from Pat and the weekly sanctioned phone calls from me. He seemed to take each new piece of news with disappointment and stoic resolve.

I found it strange to be the conduit for news shared between my sister and our family. They often passed their concerns back to her through me. Visits were restricted, and Victoria had turned inward, often too sick and exhausted to engage with the outside world. She was unable to handle anyone else's anxiety and fear; she had more than enough of her own to contend with. She was also saving her reserves for Pat and her boys.

Her days were consumed with the administration of medications and chasing the side effects. As is often the case with prolonged hospitalizations, day and night get confused and sleep becomes fitful and sporadic. She received steroids to combat possible rejection after her transplant, but these made sleep difficult. She was often awake during the night, adding to a growing sense of isolation and disengagement from her "real" life. As the transplant progressed, she faced engraftment syndrome, developing a deep red rash over her chest. Each night, her fevers would spike as high as 103°. Her lungs filled with fluid and she resorted to supplemental oxygen when she became short of breath. Feverish, disoriented, and depleted, my sister was confined to her room for the first thirty days following her transplant. These were her darkest hours.

At last, on day thirty-nine, a brutally hot day in May, Victoria was well enough to be discharged to a rental home in Pasadena, a short drive from the hospital in the event she became acutely ill. She would not be permitted to return home to Santa Monica for 100 days post-transplant. Her family moved into the rental, settling for what would be their summer holidays. Caroline and my mother, as well as several close friends, took turns staying in the house overlooking the mountains. Each guest was trained in the protocols of keeping a sterile home: wiping door handles, keeping the windows sealed, cleaning the house, and preparing safe meals. The fresh vegetables and salad Victoria craved were not allowed. Nor were raw fish or fruits without peels. Mostly, she ate cooked vegetables and prepared meals.

Those weeks coupled joy at being united with her family and tremendous fatigue. She still had to restrict contact with people, always wearing a mask and rarely venturing outdoors. Many things we take for granted are not possible after bone marrow transplant. Fresh food can carry potentially lethal bacteria. You cannot venture into public places or parks with grasses and pollens. Even though Victoria was free from the confines of the hospital, she was weak and bloated from all the medications and intravenous fluids, stuck indoors with a mask. She had frequent bouts of diarrhea and still suffered from shortness of breath.

> I'm out! Free. Good Lord, I've got gratitude growing in every cell. I wish I was able to be at home, and yet the house Pat found is very peaceful. It seems like a good place in which to continue to heal. Big picture windows and mountain and golf course views. Very comfortable bed, comfortable couch and chairs, and comfortable deck, which is slightly less appealing given that I must wear a mask at all times when outside.
>
> And they have been very discouraging about the sun. Apparently, I have the immune system and the skin of a newborn. Another year of this. Such a long journey.   —MAY 15, 2015

Still, she had made it to the other side of the transplant and there was reason to be hopeful. A bone marrow biopsy performed shortly before discharge from City of Hope showed that Nick's cells had taken over and that there were no signs of leukemic cells lurking. She was still taking steroids and an antirejection drug called tacrolimus, in addition to pain medication (oxycodone) on a regular basis for generalized bodily pains. The graft-versus-host rash was unpleasant and associated with severe itching, especially on her chest.

As Victoria grew stronger, she was able to walk one or two miles on a treadmill. She played board games with her sons and found a quiet place to rest next to one of the large picture windows. She had a view of the distant brown foothills of the mountains, which must have been inspiring. She laughed and giggled with her boys, relishing seeing them each day.

Victoria was beginning to understand the chronic nature of her disease and the regime of tests and drugs. While in Pasadena, she returned to City of Hope twice weekly for blood tests, ingesting a staggering number of pills each day. She texted me: "Wish my stuff had more of a clear ending. I'll adjust, but it's a bit crushing to think winning the war doesn't necessarily mean ending the issues. Longing to be done and return to normal. Guess there will be a new normal." Unfortunately, this is a conclusion at which many of my own patients arrive when managing a brain tumor or other types of cancer.

> Stage IV. The bizarre thing is that I'm still bargaining for my own survival. Statistically speaking, we can't all make it. Sometimes I wonder if I was slow to socialize because I was feeling dreadful and people look scary behind their masks, or was I too afraid to make a friend in case I had to hear they didn't make it? I need to work on this.
>
> I'm here and I'm staying here. I am one of the miracles, and I thank the heavens for my village for making it so. I've got this. What is this "strength" I have of which so many people speak? I don't feel strong, but

I do have blinders on—one goal only, which is to be fine. I suppose this makes every single moment of upheaval easier, because no matter how hard the moments can be (and this is an understatement), if it's just today's challenge on the way to the goal, then you just do it, you just get through it!

Any one of these enormous challenges could have slayed me, but instead, you just do what needs to be done—ride out the 103° fever, being packed on ice! Then test after test. I've fluid in the lungs, the rash, the itching—you just go through it because it's the way to recovery.

I request a most benevolent outcome that the miracles continue in my recovery from my illness.

I request that my donor cells calm down and cease attacking my skin or anything else,* realizing they are in a safe environment and all is well. (*Except for any future cancerous cells, which they are encouraged to obliterate.)

I therefore request that the GVHD [graft-versus-host disease] calm down, and that I be treated and weaned off all my medicines!

I request that I feel increasingly like myself! And that I have no ongoing residual challenges or side effects.

I request perfect health and excellent energy.

I request a continued miracle in health that is better than anyone could ever hope for or expect.

And I am overflowing with gratitude for the help, the support, the love, that has gotten me this far. Thank you!

So glad Pat is here. So, so glad. Can't stay awake, but so glad. Grateful.

—MAY 29, 2015

July. Day 82.

It's a weepy place to live when you see joy everywhere.

I am feeling so happy. I am very shaky from the medicine changes but feeling great and happy. Tired of my same psychology. I feel more like a patient today, but I don't care. I'm waking up way too early again. But yesterday and today, I had the nicest time working and playing with my boys. I love them so much.   —JULY 1, 2015

Happy 4th! A holiday where I'm with my family, not at Saint John's or City of Hope. How great is that? I'm reading Dr. Bernie Siegel's *Love, Medicine and Miracles*. I weep on almost every page, as it all resonates so deeply with me.

My tears are those of recognition that, yes, I am one of [Siegel's] "exceptional patients." I came upon this all on my own. I was a sponge for all that wisdom, for meditation, visualization, for self-empowerment—

anything that would assist me in obliterating my cancer, learning from it, fully embarking on my life and my loves.

I've never thought of myself as spiritual. I've waited on reading any numbers predicting my future. I've always known that I would be okay.

Yes, there have been moments of fear—how could there not be?—but in my heart, I know I'm fine and that I will live a long and joy-filled life.

I choose life and joy and love. Death is not an option.   —JULY 4, 2015

At about day sixty-five, Victoria's platelet count began to drop. The last time she checked, it was 231,000, which is normal. A normal count would be in the range of 150,000 to 450,000. Less than a week later, her count fell to 136,000. By July 9, her platelets had dropped to 90,000. Dr. O'Donnell decreased the antirejection drugs, hoping this would reverse the slide, but the measure didn't seem to have any effect. On July 14, Victoria's platelet count plummeted to 54,000. She received a four-hour infusion of immunoglobulin (IVIG) in the hope that this would encourage her count to rebound. While Dr. O'Donnell had indicated the decline in platelets could be from drug reactions, she did not mention to any of us that Victoria's leukemia might have returned, as a dropping platelet count is one of the first signs. This, it turned out, was indeed the case. On July 17, Victoria's platelet count dipped down to 41,000. A peripheral blood count revealed a return of blasts, now as high as 20 percent.

The leukemia was back and with a vengeance. Previously, 100 percent of Victoria's bone marrow cells were from Nick; now that number was at 90 percent, and the remaining 10 percent of the white cells in her blood contained her own DNA. These were the cells from her original leukemia, which had survived all the brutal chemotherapy, the whole-body radiation, and the bone marrow transplant. They were roaring back to life, seemingly unscathed. Dr. O'Donnell pressed on, starting my sister on a new type of chemotherapy called decitabine, with the aim of keeping regrowth of her leukemia in check. They could no longer treat her with new or potent chemotherapy drugs given the tenuous hold of her transplanted cells.

Aggressive treatment would kill off these newly arising cells and, with them, Victoria.

A week later, she texted me: "I'm scared, my brother. But I still feel determined and strong. I'm not going down with this crappy disease. Not an option. Not how I expected to spend Day 97 . . . Think good thoughts for me, and please tell everyone all I want to hear is how strong I am and how I'm going to beat this again, but for good." That night, after they cut back her immunosuppressing drugs in the hope of stimulating graft-versus-host attack of Nick's transplanted cells against the resurgent leukemia, Victoria spiked a fever to 102.3°.

On day ninety-nine, just before the long-awaited discharge home, Victoria was back in the hospital. "Doing so-so, to be honest. Definitely freaked by new development, and achy too. I will not accept defeat, but I am scared." She was admitted through the ICU and started on broad antibiotics for high fevers and a bladder infection. Her fevers rose as high as 103.5°.

I texted her back: "You inspire me. I am trying to bring your positive attitude and courage to my patients. It is very helpful."

She replied: "I could see being beaten down from this, and I see how some of those people don't make it. That's not an option for me. I've read a lot of inspirational books I can share with you. Do you know Dr. Bernie Siegel? He has some useful things to say."

By this point, the fevers were beginning to trend down, but the blast count was hovering around 36 percent. They sent her home after the first round of the new chemotherapy to get some rest and to have a break from her seemingly interminable hospitalization.

I remember saying to my wife, when Victoria broke the news over the phone that her leukemia had returned, "There is no way out of this." Yet people were rallying, digging in for a second battle.

On a return visit to City of Hope, Victoria's platelet count had decreased to 13,000. One morning, she thought she was the recipient of a miracle when her blood test came back with 0 percent blasts, but when the test was repeated, the numbers showed 37 percent. The miraculous absence of her leukemic cells was most likely only the result of a laboratory error. She completed her second ten-day cycle of decitabine at home in Santa Monica, and her blasts gradually came down to 24 percent. The idea was to put her into a less acute state, a sort of chemo limbo land, where she would live until a better strategy arose.

Victoria began throwing up on September 5 and was running fevers from 100° to 103°. "Feel horrible . . . this is so old," her text read. On the eighth: "Turns out I have sepsis. Bacteria in my blood. But feel much better after steroids. Need to raise my blood pressure. Jeez. What a thing."

She had been readmitted to the ICU in septic shock and was administered Neo-Synephrine, a powerful blood-pressure-supporting intravenous infusion. They changed her PICC line but felt that the sepsis was from E. coli. Victoria rebounded from the septic shock on broad-spectrum antibiotics and blood pressure support. Her liver tests were elevated, suggesting organ damage as a result of the sepsis incident. Her low blood pressure during the episode of sepsis and the resulting poor perfusion of circulating blood to her organs was the likely cause.

That weekend, Pat took Nick and twelve friends out for Nick's sixteenth birthday. Victoria was stuck in the hospital, but she looked forward to the boys visiting before the sleepover party. She was determined to make it back home as planned early that next week. This was her tenth month of being critically sick; she missed her family desperately. The following Monday, Pat would make the long drive back to City of Hope after he dropped Nick and Will at school. His hands were full with a bunch of teenage boys over the weekend, camped out on the floor of their den, slumbering late into Sunday morning.

Victoria was starting to feel better, despite spiking fevers greater than 103.5°. Because of my sister's general improvement, Dr. O'Donnell moved her from the ICU to a regular room, with plans to discharge her home in the next few days. She wanted Victoria's fevers to abate, with the plan of administering home intravenous antibiotics through her new PICC line.

Late Sunday night, I texted: "Good luck with all that. I'm thinking a lot about you."

She replied: "Thanks."

"Hang in there, Toria," I responded. I didn't realize that my wife had sent a series of texts to Victoria earlier that evening. They were talking about Nick's party and how the silver lining might have been that she was also going to miss the cleanup part of it. "Guess so. I'm okay, just tired of it all."

The next day, while I was seeing patients in my office, Pat sent me a text: "Sit down. Victoria passed away this morning. Totally unexpected. Please tell your family. I am going home to tell the boys."

Victoria was beginning to feel better after her episode of septic shock. She was regaining her appetite and had eaten her breakfast. At 7 a.m., the nurse came to administer her scheduled medications, which my sister took without difficulty. When the nurse came back to check on her, she was unresponsive. They called a code and did CPR, but they were unable to resuscitate her. She was pronounced dead shortly thereafter.

Less than six months earlier, Victoria had written

> Such an odd state I'm in. I feel like I am treading water, neither here nor there. . . . Being outdoors, breathing fresh air, feeling the sun beating down on me, listening to the occasional splash in the pool and the constant flow of the fountain at my right. Life is very good, very sweet here, indeed and all I want is more of it. Life. Sweetness. More sun, more breeze, more joy.
>
> —MARCH 26, 2015

When Victoria's leukemia returned so early after transplant, she was doomed. A search of the literature on survival rates after early recurrence of AML (defined as being within six months of transplant) quotes 95 percent mortality within one year. Others cite a 4 percent three-year survival after early relapse. Victoria had an extremely early recurrence at two to three months posttransplant. The new chemotherapy was a temporizing measure. Dr. O'Donnell spoke of new protocols and experimental treatments, but in truth, they had very little left to offer. My sister's best shot for survival had been transplant. When that failed, there weren't any other good options.

Dr. O'Donnell explained that Victoria had likely died of a cardiac arrhythmia brought on by damage to her heart muscle as the result of low blood pressure from the episode of septic shock. This was unforeseen but was also not preventable. The morning of her death, Pat was stunned and felt that he hadn't seen it coming. He asked me whether an autopsy would be useful, but on speaking with Dr. O'Donnell it didn't seem that it would yield any useful information, so we did not request that one be performed.

In many ways, I am glad that my sister did not know that she was about to die. She was spared a prolonged decline into disability in which decisions to abandon treatment would have needed to be made. But her reluctance to face the implications behind her leukemia's return denied her an opportunity to discuss the possibility of death with her family or the chance to express specific concerns and wishes. Because everyone was intent on cure and survival, her death came as a shock, whereas in reality, death was the most likely outcome. I'm sure that Dr. O'Donnell knew this, but I imagine she was torn.

Was it her job to confront Victoria with the prospect of death, and a death that was fairly imminent, thereby extinguishing my sister's hope for survival? If it weren't for the arrhythmia, would Victoria still be alive today? This, too, gives rise to other questions. At what cost? Even with survival from leukemia, in the best of circumstances, Victoria would have been at risk for secondary malignancies, not to mention the risk for infections arising from her weakened immunity. At this point, however, she was unlikely to survive at all, given her early recurrence after transplant. I suspect that Dr. O'Donnell would have begun to delicately map out the reality of Victoria's predicament once further treatment did not produce results, and perhaps Victoria and her family would have had the opportunity to say their meaningful goodbyes.

I called to thank Dr. O'Donnell shortly after Victoria's death. She and I both cried, each of us feeling our own pain and a profound sense of defeat. I had lost my sister; Dr. O' Donnell had lost her patient. She had done everything she could to cure Victoria, but in the end her efforts had not been enough. We simply are not yet there on the frontier of cancer cures and medicine.

I have been there many times myself: for all the new technology in the operating rooms and the best of intentions, I frequently come up short. While I know it is the cancer we are fighting and that ultimately results in death, it is hard not to take this failure personally. Just as Pat and his family were running "what-ifs" through their heads, so, too, were Victoria's doctors and medical teams. At this point, despite all our knowledge and efforts, we are often powerless to solve some intractable problems or to reverse terrible illnesses. It is our hope that a cure for this form of leukemia will be found. Childhood leukemia used to be a universal killer, but now it is one of the great cancer success stories. I can only hope that the same gains will be made in the treatment of acute leukemia in adults and in other aggressive forms of cancer.

I was thinking back to a day not so long ago (well, preleukemia), probably last October—I was at one of my kids' soccer games and someone came over, said hello, and asked how I was and how my acting career was going. It was actually going extremely well and I felt so happy!

I was about to get things moving again (ironically, right when this happened), but I didn't say anything like that—instead, I found myself laughing since I was literally sitting right next to Jodie Foster (a completely lovely devoted fellow mom at my kids' Westside LA school). I just found myself thinking of that moment and realizing I am forever altered by what

I've just experienced. In a world where a beautiful twenty-seven-year-old dies from this nasty disease, I am in the fight of my life. And glaringly confident that I am making it. But it's the same world where a fellow seventh grade mom just died of thyroid cancer. I didn't realize that could kill you. I'm in that world, and I realize that someone's celebrity—which used to intimidate me—is so unimportant. When people are capable of such love and generosity in helping my family, none of that seems to matter. I certainly don't care anymore. You're more successful, you're less successful, it's all so random anyway. Some of the most talented people I know never did all that well. It's all so unimportant to me now.   —MAY 15, 2015

Two hundred and fifty people came to pay their respects to my sister and her family at Casa del Mar in Santa Monica nearly a month after her death. The memorial was nondenominational, although there were references to Judaism, Catholicism, and Buddhism made during the service. A fellow City of Hope patient who had successfully undergone bone marrow transplantation himself made his way to the stage. His name was Bob, and to most of us he was a complete stranger. He looked frail as he stepped up to the microphone, but his brave act was not lost on any of us. He spoke in a quiet voice, deferential and full of great respect for our family.

"Perhaps I knew Victoria for a shorter time than anyone else here. I met with her and Pat for a few hours, encouraging her about her upcoming bone marrow transplant at City of Hope. I, too, had AML leukemia and a transplant at the City of Hope. I said there were ways of negotiating the protocols, like how they wanted to wake you up at 4:30 a.m. to ask how well you were sleeping. 'I was sleeping just fine, until you woke me up!' I pointed out. I had them put a sign on the door: 'Do not wake until 8:00 a.m.'

"During those few hours I met with Victoria, I was impressed by her positive attitude, her warmth, and her spirit. She was a *shtarker*, and for those of you who don't know Yiddish, it means a fighter, someone you don't mess with.

"She reminded me of a character from the play *Our Town*. Emily is a young woman who has died in childbirth and is looking down on the significant moments of her life from the beyond. 'It goes by so fast, we don't even have time to look at one another. Does anybody on earth realize how beautiful life is, while they're living it? Every, every moment?' Now, that's tough, because there are lots of annoying moments. But maybe if we think of Victoria, we can have more moments of grace and generosity and strength."

I walked out of the hotel and onto the terrace at Casa del Mar, drenched in bright sunlight, the long blue-gray horizon of the Pacific beyond. I took a deep breath of air, appreciating the scene all the more when I thought how my sister would never experience these simple joys again. In the rush of our daily lives we take these gifts for granted, or worse, reduce them to irritations and distractions. Traffic, abrasive people, unanswered messages, deadlines. What my sister would have given to be walking barefoot in the sand, inhaling the sharp, salty air!

Back in the ballroom, Victoria's warm and graceful spirit brought the speakers together. Her friends filled the room with anecdotes, memories, reflections, laughter, and tears. Kathleen Marshall, a classmate from Smith and herself a theater director and producer, reminisced about their college days:

"Victoria, as we all know, had many talents beyond her extraordinary acting ability. Most of all, she was a connector, a conduit for all of her friends and family. How many of us here have met someone through Victoria who then became an important part of our lives? How many of us who have never even met before today can say, 'Oh, I know who you are—I've heard Victoria talk about you'? With Victoria it was barely one degree of separation. She was always figuring out ways to connect people and was always thinking of others, almost more than she thought of herself: 'You should read this book,' 'You should meet this person,' 'You should take this class,' 'You should go for that job.' Toria's fierce loyalty and devotion to her friends is legendary. And her unwavering

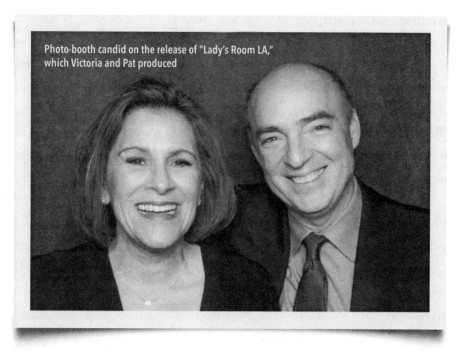

Photo-booth candid on the release of "Lady's Room LA," which Victoria and Pat produced

faith in our ability to do anything we wanted made us believe that we actually could."

Pat recounted their early relationship: "I have never met a more generous artist. Victoria took as much joy from a friend landing a part as she did when she got work. Victoria never liked it much, but I often told her she'd make a great agent because she was more dedicated to advancing other people's careers than her own.

"Even though her career never hit the big time, Victoria was happy. She told me she was happy many times, and I couldn't think of a better thing to hear her say.

"What has the last year been like? As we learned firsthand, leukemia is not for sissies. But Victoria was incredibly brave and upbeat, even in the face of extreme adversity. Our boys were Victoria's constant motivation. Her hospital room was covered with their pictures. Those pictures were always the first things to go up and the last thing to come down.

"Victoria and I certainly shed more than a few tears when she was first diagnosed. But after that, what made us choke up the most were the seemingly unlimited acts of kindness from so many of you. What our family was going through definitely took the support of a village.

"So many of you chipped in with meals, the driving, playdates, sleepovers and many gifts for our boys, and everything imaginable to make Victoria more comfortable. Many people canceled vacations, used their days off from work, and put their own lives on hold for weeks at a time to help care for Victoria, me, Nick, and Will. You have all been amazing. Thank you."

Pat went on to address his two sons: "This is and will continue to be very hard for each of us. Frankly, Mom is irreplaceable. But she was a valiant and brave fighter, and we need to try to be the same. Mom was always so positive and convinced that she would beat her leukemia that we never had an opportunity to say goodbye. That is too bad. I know she would have written each of you the longest letters telling you how much she loved you, how proud she was of you, and how honored she was to be your mom.

"In time, each of us needs to strive to live the full life that Mom would want. She'd want us to laugh, to be happy, to have fun, to take risks, to have adventures, just as if she was still here.

"I believe Mom would say to both of you, 'Always try new things. Say yes when something new or different or hard or challenging comes along. It's okay if you fail. In fact, fail a lot, as that means you are stretching yourself. Always be curious and learn new things. Go places you've never been, meet new people. If you stick to your dreams and don't give up, you can do anything.'

"And of course, being Mom, she'd also have added: 'Turn off that video game and go outside and play . . . and practice your musical instruments. And don't forget to put the toilet seat down.'

"A friend recently wrote me something beautiful that stuck with me," Pat concluded. "'Victoria will be greatly missed, but also greatly remembered, and she lives on in the memories of all those who knew her or who she touched or influenced in any way.'"

CHAPTER SEVEN

pat
(also a love story)

> It is a curious thing, the death of a loved one. We all know that our time in this world is limited, and that eventually all of us will end up underneath some sheet, never to wake up. And yet it is always a surprise when it happens to someone we know. It is like walking up the stairs to your bedroom in the dark and thinking there is one more stair than there is. Your foot falls down, through the air, and there is a sickly moment of dark surprise as you try and readjust the way you thought of things.
>
> —LEMONY SNICKET, *HORSERADISH*

> Alison and I also talked about how this ("this" being the book, the play, whatever comes from this, because something must) is also a love story. I suppose that is true. I *cannot* imagine doing this without Pat or my amazing loving boys and friends. I told Pat that as scared as I am about the upcoming transplant, I know that I can get through it with him at my side.
>
> —FEBRUARY 23, 2015

I texted Pat to wish him a happy Father's Day and to let him know I was almost done with writing the book. He had just returned from a whirlwind college tour with his boys. They had purchased a Mercedes sprinter van, which they drove between colleges in the Midwest as if they were fraternity brothers on a road trip. I asked Pat if he wanted to see the finished manuscript, uncertain about his reaction because he hadn't read Victoria's journals. I wasn't sure he would be able to face them. He texted back: "I am grateful and impressed that you have finished it. Instead of getting a copy now, how about you sign a copy for me and send it once it gets published?"

Three weeks later, I announced to Kathryn that I had finally finished writing, just shy of two years after Victoria's death. Out for dinner with friends that same night, we received an urgent call from an intensive care physician at UCLA Medical Center. Pat had been brought in by ambulance. He was in a coma and on a ventilator. The doctor explained that Pat had collapsed after a workout with Nick; he'd become unresponsive and stopped breathing. Nick had been home alone with his father at the time. He'd had the presence of mind to call 9-1-1 and start CPR. Paramedics inserted a breathing tube into Pat's trachea and took him to the UCLA Medical Center in Westwood.

An emergent head CT showed that my brother-in-law had a subarachnoid hemorrhage, most likely caused by a ruptured aneurysm, which filled the undersurface of his brain with blood. Indeed, a CT angiogram showed a small blister on the anterior communicating artery, which connects the two carotid arteries. This was felt to be the likely source of his hemorrhage. The anterior communicating artery forms the front portion of the circle of Willis at the base of the brain, which ensures redundancy of blood supply but is often a site of weaknesses in arteries, whose walls can balloon to form aneurysms.

In addition to extensive bleeding, Pat developed obstructive hydrocephalus, a condition in which the fluid chambers, or ventricles, inside the brain become enlarged and exert pressure on the surrounding brain. This can cause coma and, if untreated, rapidly lead to death. Normally, spinal fluid is produced inside the brain, circulates in the subarachnoid space, is reabsorbed into the veins along the top of the brain, and serves to provide a protective cushion for the brain. A subarachnoid hemorrhage fills this space with blood and blocks the normal circulation of cerebrospinal fluid.

Years before, Pat underwent two surgeries to repair a faulty heart valve. This congenital malformation of his aortic valve is known as a bicuspid ("two-leaves") valve, instead of the normal tricuspid, or three-leaflet, aortic valve. There is an association between this condition and the formation of brain aneurysms, but a screening scan of his brain from 2010 was normal. Before his valve replacement, his aortic valve was stiffer than normal, causing severe aortic stenosis, restricting normal blood flow from his heart. This would cause heart failure if left untreated. The first replacement had used a pig valve, which does not require blood thinners. But an infection of the valve soon after his first surgery caused rapid deterioration of the replacement; within ten years he required a second surgery. This second surgery had been technically difficult because of scarring on his heart against the inside of his chest.

At the time, his surgeons had chosen to install a mechanical aortic valve instead of a bioprosthetic one, the logic being that mechanical valves typically last longer. They had hoped this would allow him to avoid the bleeding risk of a third surgery. The downside of a mechanical valve is that the patient needs to be on anticoagulation with warfarin or Coumadin for the rest of his life. Without a strong blood thinner, the turbulent blood flow leads to thrombus, or clot formation, which can cause a stroke. Ever since his second heart surgery, Pat had needed to check his blood clotting and adjust his daily Coumadin dosing to keep his blood thin enough to prevent a stroke.

Pat had always been athletic and loved to ride a road bicycle. He had to severely cut back on risky activities because any fall or injury could cause dangerous internal bleeding. But even without an accident, bleeding is often much worse for a person on blood thinners, particularly in the brain. This was the case with his aneurysm rupture. While protective of his heart, the thinned blood likely contributed to a greater amount of blood leakage from the ruptured aneurysm, evidenced by a thicker and more extensive blood clot at the base of Pat's brain. In addition to a more severe hemorrhage, the doctors at UCLA were unable to treat his hydrocephalus until the effect of the blood thinner was reversed. Once it was safe to treat the hydrocephalus, a flexible drainage tube was placed by Dr. Patel, a neurosurgical trainee, without difficulty.

SUNDAY

I spoke at length with Dr. Patel at 2:30 on Sunday morning before driving an hour from Greensboro to Raleigh to board yet another flight to Los Angeles at 7:00 a.m. Dr. Patel explained that their preference would be to coil the aneurysm (a procedure done with catheters from within a patient's blood vessel), but given the anatomy of the aneurysm (small, no neck), they would not be able to do this with coils. Instead, they would have to clip the aneurysm surgically.

As the only physician in the extended family, I was asked by Pat's family to make medical decisions on his behalf. I reviewed the options with them and consented to craniotomy and surgical clipping of the aneurysm, which was to start that morning.

The surgical treatment of an aneurysm does not improve a patient's neurologic condition, but it does prevent additional, potentially life-threatening hemorrhages from occurring. Eliminating the aneurysm also allows doctors to treat late complications of subarachnoid hemorrhage, such as vasospasm. This causes constriction of the arteries supplying blood to the brain and can result in a stroke. Raising the patient's blood pressure will counteract vasospasm, but this is only possible if the aneurysm has been removed from the circulation, since high blood pressure will increase the risk of additional bleeding from an unsecured aneurysm. The extent of initial hemorrhage correlates with the likelihood of developing vasospasm. In Pat's case, given the large initial blood clot, later vasospasm was likely. The window for surgery in such a case is only a few days, since the risks of surgery after vasospasm has commenced are prohibitive (this typically begins four days after initial hemorrhage). So, it was now or never.

Yet, I hesitated to agree. Pat's neurologic condition was poor, and I knew, from previous discussions with him as a result of Victoria's illness and death, that he would not want to survive in a vegetative state. I was leery of setting down a procedurally driven road of surgery, tracheostomy, PEG (feeding tube), and shunt, followed by transfer to a skilled nursing facility and a potential existence, rather than a life, in long-term care. I knew he would not want that. He wanted to be there for his children, not to become a burden to them, but he would rather be dead if he could not remain vital.

It was not immediately possible to determine the cause of his diminished level of responsiveness. His initial neurologic exam was extremely poor, reflecting a deep coma (fixed, nonreactive right pupil and minimal withdrawal of his extremities to noxious stimuli, such as nail-bed pressure, but otherwise complete unresponsiveness). He would not open his eyes and would not breathe without the support of a respirator. Time would tell if he would recover from the placement of the external ventricular drain (EVD), but there was also urgency to controlling the aneurysm. By the time I boarded the plane for LA, he had not improved at all. It was worrisome that his level of coma reflected a more permanent injury, but only five hours had elapsed since the procedure. This was not long enough to know if the drain would ultimately prove effective.

There were three possible explanations for Pat's neurologic condition. The first, likely irreversible, was from the hemorrhage itself. Arterial blood released suddenly into the brain from a ruptured blood vessel can cause great damage, cutting through delicate structures like a knife through soft butter. He had presented with a devastating hemorrhage, Hunt and Hess grade four out of a possible five. Grade five means the patient is close to death. Grade one means the patient is neurologically intact except for a headache. An aneurysm rupture is like an explosion in the brain: there is direct brain injury as a result. Often, this injury is not recoverable.

The second possible explanation for his poor performance was obstructive hydrocephalus. Often, placing an EVD into the brain can reverse neurologic deterioration and people can thereafter make dramatic recoveries.

A third possibility was the period of respiratory arrest that preceded Nick's initiation of CPR. A prolonged period of oxygen deprivation could certainly cause devastating and irreversible brain injury on its own and also compound the effects of the hemorrhage and hydrocephalus.

An additional concern was that once a craniotomy has been performed, or for that matter, when there is an unsecured aneurysm, it is unsafe to resume blood thinners for at least one to two weeks. Yet throughout that period Pat would be at high risk for a stroke, which could by itself kill him. These are examples of some of the complex concerns I had and the untenable balances that needed to be struck with the chain of events unleashed by Pat's aneurysm rupture.

I talked to Dr. Patel for almost twenty minutes, both of us speaking the same medical language and having intimate familiarity with the complexities and pitfalls of managing subarachnoid hemorrhages. I explained that I was fine with proceeding with surgery but said that we would need to assess Pat's progress afterward to decide whether to continue or withdraw care. Dr. Patel indicated that this was a reasonable approach and said that the attending surgeon, Dr. Lekovic, was very compassionate and would be comfortable addressing those issues with us after Pat's surgery.

We wanted to give Pat every possible chance to recover, yet we didn't want to condemn him to a persistent vegetative state. The window of time to withdraw care is a narrow one. After the custodial procedures of shunt, feeding tube, and tracheostomy insertion have been performed, the decision to withdraw care becomes a much more uncomfortable prospect, presenting difficult choices, such as cessation of nutrition or refraining from treating incidental infections with antibiotics, and potentially causing greater suffering for the patient. If Pat did not make progress after surgery, he would still be dependent on the ventilator and the EVD, and the decision to back off on those supportive measures would lead him to die peacefully and unaware of his circumstances. I knew this was the decision he would have made for himself. This is the decision I would make for myself if I were in his situation.

Some would challenge that withdrawing support would actively lead to Pat's death and deprive him of the hope of recovery. I would argue the opposite. The machines were the unnatural things keeping Pat alive. The decision to withdraw support does not condemn someone to death. Rather, it removes our mechanical interventions from condemning the person to a prolonged life of pain, lack of awareness, and suffering. Where some would cling to hope, I clung to dignity. I knew Pat would never want the marginal existence we would inflict upon him by doing all of these procedures. Putting him through such interventions would only make sense if there were a significant likelihood of his recovering consciousness and independent function.

But what of his children? Weren't they reason enough to persevere? After all, Victoria hadn't hesitated to accept whatever therapies were suggested to her, embracing them so that she could survive for her children. Even in the best-case scenario, the father whom the boys knew and loved no longer existed. Keeping Pat's body alive would not preserve him, and over time their memories of the active, passionate man they knew and loved would be supplanted by memories of visiting Pat in a nursing home, of bedsores, urinary tract infections, and contractures, of their father physically wasting away. It was devastating to realize that my nephews, in the space of two years, would become orphans. I worried that Nick probably felt guilt and personal failure, while I saw only devotion and heroism. On two separate occasions he acted with tremendous maturity and courage on behalf of his parents, the first time as a willing stem cell donor for his mother's bone marrow transplant and the second by calling 9-1-1 and initiating CPR, alone, on his father.

In the end, despite all our knowledge and skill, we are frequently powerless to undo that which has befallen us. Recognizing our limitations, we must cure when we can and console when we cannot, all the while being as honest and empathetic as possible. We must be willing to accept defeat and discontinue treatment, admitting our limitations. This is often more difficult than continuing in pursuit of long odds and unrealistic hope, as so often happens in ICUs and acute care settings, where efficiency of care is often valued and tough decisions may be deferred.

I met Joe Whelan, one of Pat's older brothers, his wife Deanna, and Diane, a close family friend, at the hospital. By the time I arrived on that quiet Sunday morning, Pat was in surgery. A number on a screen in the first-floor surgical waiting area had gone to red, indicating the procedure had begun. After an hour of sitting with no news, I snuck past security with one of the visitors' passes and made my way to the sixth floor, the neurotrauma ICU. I pleaded my case into the security phone outside the locked double doors to the ICU. Even to a physician who understands the way hospitals work, this seemed like an intimidating and impersonal place. The charge nurse, Holly, came to the door. I explained that Joe, Deanna, and I had arrived from the East Coast and were sitting in the surgical waiting room on the main level, hoping for news. She called down and found out that the surgery had only just begun and would continue for at least six hours. With that information, she gave me a generous, empathetic hug and advised that we leave the hospital and try to get some rest. Later, she was gracious enough to call at 3:00 p.m. and let us know that we should return to the hospital around 4:30.

On our return, we were attempting to negotiate our way past security when I recognized Dr. Lekovic (I had seen his picture on the UCLA website) striding confidently across the lobby. I intercepted him and we introduced ourselves. He seemed to soften when I explained that I was also a neurosurgeon. He was pleased with how the surgery had gone but said that Pat remained critically ill. I explained that, while we wanted to give Pat every possible chance to recover, we did not want him to have a tracheostomy, PEG, or shunt placed unless he was clearly improving, as he had indicated he did not want to end up in a nursing home or remain in a persistent vegetative state.

Taken aback, Dr. Lekovic explained that there was still a good chance that Pat would recover and that they were going to do everything they could for at least the next one to two weeks. If, after that, he did not improve and regain consciousness, the surgeon agreed that we should not allow a tracheostomy to be placed, and at that point, we would draw a line and discontinue treatment. Initially, Dr. Lekovic seemed quite nervous about this line of thinking and expressed optimism that Pat might recover, but in the space of this brief but important conversation, he explained the decisions we (Joe, Deanna, and I) would need to make and the timing for making them, including the two-week limit for a temporary breathing tube before a tracheostomy would need to be performed.

MONDAY
The hospital had come to life as we returned to Pat's bedside the next morning. The Neuro-ICU nursing staff encouraged us to come to ICU rounds and to interact with the medical team. Dr. Blanco was the Neurology Intensive Care attending. Soft-spoken, thoughtful, and kind, he was also patient and informative. He and I spoke the "neuro" language, which I translated to Joe and Deanna, and later to the Whelan and Stern families in hour-long conference calls. We also met with Pat and Victoria's close friends to review his progress in another conference, this one at Diane's home. These discussions, followed by explanatory emails, took hours each day over the ensuing week, but they proved essential to helping families and friends come to understand the events that had transpired and what the future held. Without them, everyone would have felt much more in the dark.

Pat lay in bed, eyes closed, with his head elevated on a pillow. There was a bulky white bandage on his head with some bloody drainage on the right side where Dr. Lekovic and his team had opened Pat's skull. A slender white plastic EVD tube led from the bottom edge of the dressing, draining pink blood-tinged spinal fluid into a sterile collecting system, while a bundle of multicolored electrical cables, leading to an EEG monitor, emerged from the top. Pat was loosely covered with a hospital gown. His prior chest incision was plainly visible. He had an arterial line in his groin, as well as intravenous lines in both arms and a radial arterial line in his left wrist. He had multiple intravenous drips and monitors in addition to the continuous EEG monitoring, which assessed for possible seizure activity and for electrical signs of wakefulness. There were sequential compression devices on both of his legs to help prevent blood clots from forming. A CT scan and CT angiogram done early in the morning showed no surgical complications and indicated that the aneurysm was no longer filling, evidence that it had been successfully clipped.

When Dr. Blanco and his team came in, they introduced themselves and examined Pat. Pat did not open his eyes or respond to voice. He did not follow commands. His pupils were minimally reactive. He extended his arms forcefully down and away (extensor posturing) to painful stimulation and withdrew his legs (triple flexion) in response to pain. The latter is a reflex movement, while the former indicates a relatively low level of brain function and is, in itself, a form of reflex movement. The doctors had given Pat no sedation since the surgery, but they felt that his brain activity might still be suppressed by a large dose of pentobarbital, a powerful barbiturate, which had been given at the time of surgery to protect the brain from damage, since they had to temporarily block the blood flow to his brain in order to clip his aneurysm. This long-acting drug takes twelve to twenty-four hours to wear off and leave the system. The EVD seemed to be working well, but the treatment of his hydrocephalus had not appeared to improve his level of consciousness. Dr. Blanco expressed cautious optimism and suggested that with time Pat might improve, saying that for now they would hold off on making comments about his long-term prognosis.

We went home and reported to the boys, who were interested but did not want a lot of details, as this was clearly more than they were able to deal with. They played video games and mostly stayed in their rooms.

Neighbors and friends had once again begun cooking for the family; the refrigerator was stuffed with food. The blue plastic cooler filled with meals was placed on the front porch, as it had been throughout Victoria's illness. Joe and I attempted to find Pat's healthcare directives, and Joe contacted Pat's attorney, who produced a draft document that had not been executed. This draft stated that Victoria was his healthcare power of attorney, but in case of her incapacity, that role passed to my wife and me. We surmised that Pat had not rewritten the document after Victoria's death. While I had been interjecting opinions and advising the family, it now appeared that I was actually the family member appointed to make medical decisions on Pat's behalf.

TUESDAY

The next morning, we returned to the hospital and again attended rounds. Dr. Blanco and his team examined Pat. There had been no change over the past twenty-four hours apart from some worrisome EEG activity with some slowing of his brain waves, suggestive of brain damage, and some spiking activity, worrisome in that it suggested early seizure-like activity, for which they increased his Levetiracetam (antiseizure medication) dosing. By this point, the barbiturates were out of his system and his hydrocephalus had been treated, with the pressure relieved.

Pat remained deeply comatose. A cardiologist came to check on Pat and an echocardiogram was performed, showing that his heart was working fine and his mechanical valve was functioning properly.

WEDNESDAY

I had planned to fly back to North Carolina later that day. Dr. Blanco kindly came in a half hour before rounds at 7:30 a.m. to review Pat's situation with us. Pat's examination had indicated no improvement at all. He still showed no signs of responsiveness and continued to extend his upper extremities and withdraw his legs to pain. His pupils were unchanged, his gaze dysconjugate (eyes crossed, suggesting brain stem damage). He coughed, and gagged to suctioning, but otherwise did not respond to the outside world. Transcranial Doppler tests (an ultrasound probe placed against the scalp can record the velocity of blood flowing through arteries supplying the brain with blood) showed that he was developing vasospasm with increasing velocities of blood flow. Ominously, the basilar artery, which supplies the brain stem, was the artery with the greatest velocities. This was also the location of the greatest amount of hemorrhage on the CT scan obtained at Pat's initial presentation. Dr. Blanco recommended an angiogram to assess for spasm and possibly to prevent the complications of vasospasm (stroke), with an infusion of calcium channel blockers (verapamil) to counter the irritating effects of the blood on the outside of Pat's vessels.

At this point, there was a perceptible change in the outlook of the medical staff. Dr. Blanco stated that Pat's lack of improvement did not bode well for recovery. He encouraged us to continue to treat him aggressively for the next week but told us to begin to discuss with Pat's sons the possibility of withdrawing treatment should he not improve significantly. Later, Dr. Lekovic came in to meet with us and said exactly the same things. He told us that Pat had come in with a high-grade subarachnoid hemorrhage, that the treatment had been a Hail Mary pass, and that his lack of improvement did not bode well. He explained the difference between survival and a meaningful recovery.

Both doctors recommended an MRI, which would show the parts of Pat's brain that had sustained damage. This might provide useful prognostic information. We all agreed that we would give Pat until the following week to see if he improved, and that I would return to North Carolina later that day and fly back to LA the following week to consider withdrawing care and letting Pat die if there had been no improvement over that period. We felt this was most consistent with Pat's previously expressed wishes.

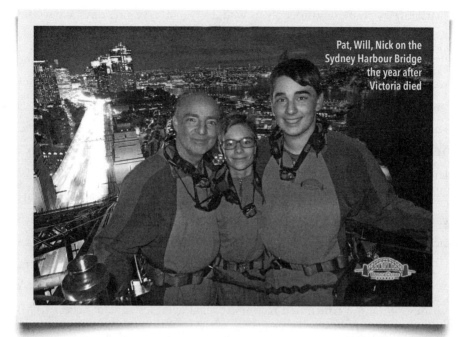

Pat, Will, Nick on the Sydney Harbour Bridge the year after Victoria died

Our hearts aching, Joe, Deanna, and I recognized that it was time to tell Nick and Will exactly what was going on. We wanted to do this before I left LA, explaining our thoughts and the plan we were putting in motion. I have told many patients and their families that they are about to die or that their loved one has already died. Yet I have never had a conversation with anyone like the conversation we had with the boys. To lose a parent is agonizing; to lose both parents in separate tragedies is almost unbearable. We want to protect our children from grim realities and from loss, but we cannot always do so.

All three adults cried as we delivered the news. The boys listened, asked a few questions, and then, surprisingly, thanked us for our honesty. Each of us knew their worlds were irreparably changed. Both boys seemed grown-up well beyond their years. We told them we would see how Pat did each day, but if he didn't improve, we would honor his wishes and not allow the three additional surgeries of tracheostomy, feeding tube placement, and implantation of a shunt. Nick and Will understood that their father did not want to end up in a nursing home and that this situation was hurting us deeply as well. In the intervening days, we would rejoice at substantive improvement but gird ourselves for its absence.

Joe drove me to the airport. We discussed the timing of the coming week: instituting a do not resuscitate (DNR) order; the assessment of Pat's progress; the involvement of palliative care services; inviting family to see Pat once more; deciding on withdrawal of care; having a graveside service. Yet another funeral. While I flew home, Joe went to Pat's bank with a letter from UCLA explaining Pat's condition with a request for access to Pat's safe deposit box in the hope that we would finally be able to locate executed advance directives, trust documents, and wills. Despite Joe's bearing a letter per Pat's lawyer's instructions, the bank denied him access to the box, so he was unable to complete his search for the documents. We decided to use the draft document as the best approximation of Pat's wishes, while Joe continued to pursue legal avenues to gain access to his safe deposit box.

I came back to Greensboro to catch up on a week of canceled patients and surgeries, but I participated in Dr. Blanco's rounds each day by speakerphone, with Joe and Deanna at Pat's bedside. At seven days after the hemorrhage, Pat remained deeply comatose. He had not improved at all and continued to extend his arms to painful stimulation with no signs of wakefulness. The medical team performed a bedside Doppler ultrasound exam that showed Pat was showering emboli, or blood clots, from his mechanical heart valve into his cerebral circulation. These would likely cause multiple small strokes but could also cause a massive one, so they started him on heparin, a blood thinner, through his IV to try to prevent this from occurring.

The next day, Pat's EEG showed some worrisome slowing over the right hemisphere, so they repeated an MRI of his brain, looking for a new stroke or hemorrhage. Dr. Blanco expressed complete agreement with continuing full support until the following Wednesday, but he also agreed that if there were no improvement, we would withdraw support Thursday evening.

There was a plan in place for a visitation, followed by a memorial service that Saturday at Woodlawn Cemetery in Santa Monica, where Victoria had a graveside burial service almost two years earlier. Notifications were sent, along with medical updates, to family members. Friends of the family offered their homes for out-of-town guests, and everyone booked flights to LA. As the week progressed, Pat's condition had not improved at all, so by Wednesday morning we were all preparing for the withdrawal of treatment.

Joe and Deanna spoke to the boys about these arrangements and asked for their opinions: burial or cremation; open or closed casket; flowers; a gathering afterward with families and friends. Nick and Will had strong opinions and appreciated being involved in the decisions. Afterward, they went over legal concepts of wills, trusts, guardianship, advance directives, and healthcare power of attorney, seeming to absorb the concepts readily. The boys decided on a memorial service immediately following Pat's funeral. Uncannily, the only venue the family could come up with on such short notice was Shutters on the Beach, which is next door to Casa del Mar, where Victoria's memorial service was held a few weeks after her burial.

Coming directly to the hospital from the airport, I met Joe and Deanna in the ICU that Wednesday morning. Dr. Vespa had replaced Dr. Blanco in the ICU. He came to Pat's bedside to speak with us. Initially, out of deference to Pat, we had conducted our discussions in the hall, away from his bed. Now, we all remained in his room. Dr. Vespa showed us Pat's MRI. He spoke of the damage to Pat's brain stem and cerebellum seen on his scan and of his lack of clinical improvement. We had an awkward discussion about the possible extent to which Pat could recover. Dr. Vespa indicated that he would almost certainly remain in a nursing home for eight-plus months, but that with improvement, it was possible that he could eventually return home—though at a minimum, he would be paralyzed on the left side of his body and he would be unlikely ever to be able to completely care for himself or regain his independence.

Although still quite bleak, this assessment was more optimistic than those provided by all the other treating physicians, an incongruity we found disquieting.

Earlier, I had asked Dr. Vespa what he would do if he were in Pat's position. He said he likely would want to be taken off life support himself. Today, however, he seemed to be cautiously offering us hope. But I pressed him. Pat had not improved at all since his admission, and his neurologic exam, despite all the tests and treatments, had not changed at all. Dr. Vespa agreed. I explained to Joe and Deanna that there was a bell-shaped curve of possible outcomes for Pat. Dr. Vespa told us that he was offering the best possible outcome, which was extremely unlikely. The most likely outcome was that Pat would never regain consciousness and would succumb to a secondary illness, such as a pneumonia, urinary tract infection, or blood clot to his lungs.

With that, we resolved to hold to our plan to invite Pat's family to see him once more and then to withdraw care the following evening at 6:00 p.m.

On Wednesday evening, the families arrived in LA and we all met for dinner at the Whelan house. I spoke with Barb, Pat's youngest sister. She and her husband, Dan were the designated legal guardians for Nick and Will. I explained the medical situation once again and answered many questions. Some family members wanted to see Pat once more while he was alive, but they wished to leave before the ventilator was withdrawn. Others wanted to be there for Pat's passing. Pat's father, Tom, a devout Catholic, and I spoke about cremation and the withdrawal of treatment and whether this was acceptable to him and to the church (it was). Joe, Deanna, Barb, and I planned the coming day. Nick wanted to see his father once more. Will did not wish to return to the hospital. Joe, Deanna, and Barb wanted to see Pat once more but wished to leave before Pat died. I volunteered to stay for Pat's death.

THURSDAY

The four of us attended morning rounds for the last time (there was no improvement in Pat's condition) and then had a two-hour meeting in the ICU conference room with the palliative care and hospice teams. Dr. Pietras asked me to summarize my understanding of the situation and our goals. He was accompanied by his team, which included the Neuro-ICU fellow, the palliative care fellow, the social worker, and the hospice social worker. They listened attentively as I articulated our understanding of the medical and social concerns, and our interpretation of Pat's wishes and how we wished to honor them. Joe, Deanna, and Barb were also present. I tried to synthesize the medical and the personal, giving voice to the religious concerns of some family members and expressing consideration for Pat and the boys, who did not ascribe to any organized religion, as well as to the fact that the boys were about to lose their last parent. I tried to strike a balance between these considerations. The team was supportive and agreed with our plan. Acting with healthcare power of attorney, I signed a stack of documents.

We spoke of the mechanics of removing support and of the desire to maintain comfort but not to hasten death. Dr. Pietras warned us that Pat might not die right away but could linger for days to weeks before he died, saying that there was an outside chance he might have to be transferred to a nursing home if he lingered. The family members looked at each other with new anxiety and dread. The funeral had already been planned for Saturday. We agreed that the service would proceed and become a celebration of Pat's life if, uncomfortably, he remained alive. I asked the medical team to clamp off his EVD that morning and to give him morphine to ensure he remained comfortable. The team agreed to both of these requests.

We went back to the Whelan house for a break, returning to the hospital at 5:00 p.m. Several family members, including Barb and Nick, had tearful private visits with Pat, after which they went home. Pat's parents, Julie and Tom, and his older brothers, Tom and Tim, along with their families, stayed. The chaplain and a priest visited and they prayed together.

The family took Communion. Rachel, Pat's nurse, had prepared and positioned Pat before everyone arrived. She had started a morphine drip at a low rate of infusion several hours earlier. At 6:00 p.m., she gave some intravenous medications to decrease Pat's oral secretions. We gathered in a circle around Pat's bedside, holding hands with each other and holding onto Pat. Everyone was weeping. At 6:15, the respiratory therapists came and, after suctioning Pat's mouth, removed his breathing tube. Several of the family members who had stepped out while the breathing tube was removed now returned to Pat's bedside, re-forming the circle.

Pat breathed sporadically and with difficulty. He made noises and sighs that sounded like his voice. Eerily, Pat seemed more awake than he had before. It was the first time in two weeks we had heard his voice, previously silenced by the breathing tube and the whooshing sounds of the ventilator. Julie and Tom hugged their son. Julie told him, "Pat, it's time to let go." Shortly afterward, Pat stopped breathing, his heart stopped beating, and he was gone.

So many people have shown our family such amazing support, generosity, kindness. Such profound beauty. Our friends have had the boys three times a week for months now, some people making the journey over and over. The school counselor offered repeatedly to bring us dinner from their parents' guild, but we always said no, because our friends had us more than covered.

I have felt the swell of our village supporting me, all of us, every step of the way. I am not sure I will ever stop weeping when I think about all the amazing kindness.

Most of all, I find myself crying because my partner in this, the man who has been with me every step of the way, my amazing darling husband, Pat, is heading back to Santa Monica today to be there for the boys as they wind down the school year. I've missed them *so* much. My lost year. So many recitals, sports matters, joys, and lows. I've just *missed* this year. Of course, as Pat pointed out, we'll be back here first thing tomorrow with the boys—so he won't be gone long. . . .

. . . I'll see Pat and the boys on the weekends, but he will no longer be my constant companion. He has sat with a mask on and plastic gloves—by my side for months now, there anytime I needed him. Helping me change, cleaning up all sorts of nasty things, just there, loving me. Pushing me to read, to take one more loop in our walk together, pushing my IV (Stalker) pole, opening the doors, and going two miles on our last walk! We are a team.

One patient's wife forever teased us, calling us "the lovebirds" as we walked. They said we've inspired them. It's Pat. He has never doubted—he said he was scared at first when I got the diagnosis but that he's never worried since.

He's just believed in me and my ability to win this battle.

I am eternally grateful, and I know *we* did this, together. I saw other couples get snippy with each other through this process—how could they not? So much can start stress—but we never did, not once. He never, ever lost his patience with me.

He knew my only job has been to save every ounce of energy for healing. While he juggles work, the boys' schedules, the nonstop communications with my well-wishers, making updates, all the while *at my side*. So today, my mom comes as the first in my new series of caregivers and Pat heads to Santa Monica—I feel such profound sorrow. Even though I'm making progress, I will miss Pat terribly.

I wonder if I will someday no longer weep when I look back on this time and how moved, impressed, grateful I've been by [or for] him? By our friends? Our village? How will I get through that first day I go back to school and see some of our village up close—how will I not weep? I guess I'll be carrying tissues for a long time. —MAY 15, 2015

Victoria's and Pat's experiences bookend many issues surrounding the end of life. Victoria's illness was prolonged; Pat's was brief. Victoria maintained consciousness and self-autonomy until the moment of her death. Pat presented in a coma and never regained consciousness. Victoria underwent treatments, which caused her harm, in an effort to control and cure her leukemia. Pat's treatments were an effort to save his life, treat a catastrophe, and allow his brain a chance to recover. Both were sudden and shocking diagnoses in otherwise relatively healthy adults. During Victoria's prolonged illness, there were many opportunities to discuss her condition and prognosis with her family and to prepare (to some extent) for her death. These opportunities did not exist in Pat's case. In neither instance were Victoria and Pat prepared for the possibility of death. The absence of planning and documents, such as executed living wills, contributed to the stress felt by everyone trying to exercise their wishes. In both cases, heroic efforts by talented, committed, compassionate medical teams ultimately did not prevail, despite concerted and heroic effort.

Subarachnoid hemorrhage and coma are disease processes with which I have great familiarity. I have spent much of my career caring for patients with aneurysm ruptures and hydrocephalus. I have counseled families, seen many patients recover, and discontinued care in others. Until Pat's illness, however, I had never found myself so closely involved in and directly responsible for decisions. I was the designated healthcare power of attorney. It was up to me, legally, to decide whether to persevere or to withdraw. I felt the weight of those decisions. I also felt powerless to effect changes in Pat's condition and could only use my knowledge to explain to his family and friends what was happening.

Because of this knowledge, I could see, more clearly than other family members, that all the interventions, from the EVD placement to the aneurysm clipping to the two weeks of waiting for Pat to improve, led to no significant change in his condition. Even though the doctors encouraged us to be hopeful, there never was cause for optimism. Pat never improved at all.

The difference between being a concerned doctor and an invested family member is huge. Conveying the details of Pat's illness to family and friends took hours each day. It included multiple conversations, conferences, and emails; reviewing anatomic diagrams; explaining tests, scans, machines, and monitors at Pat's bedside; explaining the details of his neurologic examination; and having discussions with doctors, nurses, and technicians. Our discussion with the palliative care team about the mechanics of withdrawing care took well over two hours. Many of these conversations were painful and emotionally draining, especially those with Nick and Will.

The degree of disruption for the family was also extreme. I took time away from work. Other family members set aside their jobs and commitments, found childcare, traveled across the country. This experience confirmed what I had already come to understand: there is simply not enough time for a busy doctor to address all of these concerns alone. Only with a team approach can we begin to effectively answer the questions and meet the demands of families facing such emotionally draining and disruptive crises.

Despite a mortal illness, Victoria did not discuss the possibility of dying with her family or whether she wanted to be cremated or buried. Pat appeared to have prepared documents outlining his medical wishes, but these were nowhere to be found and we did not have access to his safe deposit box. As a result of this experience, each of my children immediately sent advance directives to our attorney naming healthcare powers of attorney and stating their wishes for a natural death and cremation. My wife and I have done the same. We will make sure these documents are easily accessible.

I had been afraid to tell Nick and Will their father was going to die; but the honest and open discussions we had helped them understand and come to terms with what was happening. They rose to the occasion by being able to help plan the memorial events and the termination of life support. The family came to LA to support them, and both boys struck an inclusive and welcoming stance with all of us, which served to bring closer together the Whelans, the Sterns, and family friends.

In the end, this story is also a love story. The legacy Victoria and Pat left is one of love. They loved each other passionately. They loved life. And they loved their boys, Nick and Will. They brought people together. They taught me about how to love, how to live, and, ultimately, how to die: with preparation, acknowledgment, and, where possible, acceptance.

part
three

doctors speak: conversations with colleagues

I walked alone in the chill of dawn
while my mind leapt, as the teachers

of detachment say, like a drunken
monkey. Then a gray shape, an owl,

passed overhead. An owl is not
like a crow. A crow makes convivial

chuckings as it flies,
but the owl flew well beyond me

before I heard it coming, and when it
settled, the bough did not sway.
—JANE KENYON, "PROGNOSIS"

Having been changed as a doctor by my sister's illness and death, I began to wonder how other doctors are affected when they or a loved one fall ill. Does it change their perspective as dramatically as it changed mine? How do doctors integrate personal loss into their professional lives, and how do these experiences influence the way they relate to patients and their families? How do physicians manage their grief without withdrawing or becoming overwhelmed? How do other doctors respond when someone

129

they love does not want to hear the truth as we see it? How do they decide how much information to give their patients? How can we do better?

I decided to interview some of the doctors I know best to try to find answers to some of these questions. In the course of these interviews, I learned that we all share common experiences of loss, but that we rarely find—or make—the opportunity to discuss them with one another. As a profession, we seldom come together to express our feelings, especially when addressing failure. Physicians are expected, by ourselves and by others, to bounce back from these losses and to absorb them without consequences. This can lead to disengagement, substance abuse, early retirement, or burnout.

There is a general perception that doctors are not the same as other people. They are expected to handle difficult situations seemingly without impact. Yet physicians experience both the professional and personal sides of medical care and need to strike a balance between these areas. Just as I had to move between my medical training and practice and being a supportive older brother, the physician colleagues I interviewed have all had to balance their professional lives with their personal relationships, whether the patients are parents, spouses, aunts, or siblings, or—in one instance—when the physician was himself the patient.

I interviewed four friends and colleagues about their experiences on the "other" side of medical care. Matt Manning is a radiation oncologist whose father died of renal cancer. Gus Magrinat is an oncologist who runs our breast cancer program and whose wife, Mary, herself developed breast cancer. Stacy Wentworth is a radiation oncologist who describes the death from brain cancer of her aunt, a chief nursing officer, and the impact this had on her life, as well as her ideas about the training of physicians. Finally, I met with Sean Fischer, my sister's hematologist-oncologist, after she died, to learn his perspectives on Victoria's illness.

These community-based physicians offer perspectives and insights that are useful to us all. They also provide ideas for improving the way we render care, approach patients, and educate future physicians.

MATT MANNING

Matt is a radiation oncologist, now Chief of Oncology at Cone Health Cancer Center, who trained at the Medical College of Virginia. He moves, bear-like, through the halls of the clinic, his freshly pressed lab coat hanging on his broad shoulders. Matt's size suggests someone who might fill the room, but when he greets you (pre-coronavirus) it is often with a quiet, unassuming handshake. I have known him for twelve years and we have worked together for much of that time. Together, we convinced our hospital system to purchase a linear accelerator and begin a stereotactic radiosurgery program to treat patients with brain tumors, often instead of surgery, but also in combination with surgery.

Radiosurgery involves precisely calculating and delivering single treatments of radiation to cancerous brain tumors, which have usually spread from other organs, such as lung or breast. Matt and I created a multidisciplinary conference with a navigator, radiation oncologists, radiologists, oncologists, neurosurgeons, pathologists, geneticists, and radiation physicists to review cases on a weekly basis so that we could provide optimal care for patients. To help us address social issues affecting patients and their families, we embedded a palliative care specialist in our clinic, and we recently hired a Duke-trained neuro-oncologist to help us run and further develop the program. Over the last eight years, we have treated almost 1,000 patients.

I asked Matt what he had learned from his father's illness and death and how the experience has affected his thinking going forward. He is often optimistic about outcomes and he was so with his father, but he saw, through his father's illness, that this optimism was ill-founded. Yet previous successes with patients have helped him form this outlook and push for a successful outcome with patients, even if it seems unlikely.

As a physician with experience, if you have a number in the numerator representing success stories that you have personally been a part of, that number tends to inform decisions about your next patients. I have a couple of numbers in my numerator that will stick with me forever.

One was a case where I was working at the VA hospital as a resident in the pulmonary ICU. The VA hospital was a way station for certain patients who had critical injuries and who were on ventilators. Most were unlikely to come off the ventilator, and they spent their time in the ICU until a bed opened up in a long-term facility. One day, a guy came in who was, maybe, a thirty-five- or forty-year-old police officer. He had been injured. He was on a ventilator, and for inexplicable reasons they were never able to wean him off the ventilator. He ended up on my service.

I talked to the attending physician about different options, including treating this young guy as if he were an older end-stage smoker by allowing his CO_2 levels to rise above where we are normally comfortable. They allowed me to adjust the settings over a few days. I ended up weaning him off the ventilator, and the guy recovered and got better and went home. That is not a common scenario but having been through that experience just that one time sixteen years ago, I now look at patients on ventilators [without] feel[ing] completely hopeless.

A lung cancer patient who is ventilator-dependent often gets resigned to that being the end of their care. So, yes, I have had some experiences that make me believe that unexpected recoveries are possible, and I do not think I harm patients as a result of wanting to be more aggressive. I weigh the pros and cons of the treatments, but if you put me, an aggressive physician, with a family that wants to be optimistic but does not want a bad outcome despite the odds, our combination could be problematic. We may agree to do aggressive things, such as more courses of radiation than people might recommend or more intense chemotherapy than most patients want to endure. What could have transpired sort of peacefully over a few weeks or a month may get stretched out to a six- or eight-month period of time spent in a cancer center or in a hospital.

I get the sense from some patients that they want that time, but I think in some ways, I will mature more as a physician and potentially be less aggressive with age. I guess that may happen as I think about the experience I had with my dad and seeing the devastating consequences of dying in the ICU. As my family members age and as I become personally involved in more of these experiences on the family side, I think that it could change the way I practice.

Here, Matt's experience echoes my own. I have also become less aggressive with age and am much more motivated to avoid a protracted demise in the ICU than to chase the infinitesimal chance of recovery in a profoundly ill patient with a poor prognosis. Matt learned firsthand, through his experience with his father, the pitfalls of chasing remote possibilities of recovery.

At that age, I probably would not have had surgery done and would have gone forward with systemic treatments. There are some good ones for renal cell cancer now. Immunotherapy. You usually survive longer if you take the kidney out. I might have calculated that it was not worth the risk to go through the procedure. I would not want a feeding or a trach tube placed in me. If things were that bleak, I would not have made those same decisions.

When he [my father] went to see his urologist to talk about the scan result, his urologist recommended surgery to take the kidney out. I set aside what was a realistic, experienced recommendation in my head for what my dad ought to do, and essentially fell into this optimism of *Well, if his urologist thinks he is healthy enough to undergo this procedure, then maybe he is. Certainly, there are men in his age group who survive that and do well.*

He was seventy-six and he had had atrial fibrillation and was on anticoagulation, so there were some risks, but nephrectomy, kidney removal, is not the most challenging surgery. It is not usually a very difficult recovery, and so I went along with that decision. And I thought, *This is great if we can be as aggressive as we would be with a fifty-year-old.*

Unfortunately, my dad was pretty fearful about surgery and did not really want to do it unless I thought it was a good idea for him. I found myself falling into the same patterns of behavior that I see from my patients and their families, where you let hope drive your thinking more than realism.

The procedure turned out to be a disaster.

Dad had postoperative complications where he was bleeding internally. He had to stay off of his anticoagulation meds for several days, and the bleeding finally stopped. He was transfused probably a dozen units of blood over a few days, and then when he was starting to make a recovery, he developed a thrombus or a blood clot in his heart, and then that broke off and caused a massive stroke of the dominant side of his brain. He lost consciousness. And this is where, in talking with colleagues who were familiar with brain injury, I realized how significant this was.

Initially, I was hopeful that things may turn around, but as days went by and he did not regain consciousness, my family faced some difficult questions. You ask, "Can he recover from this? Can he get better and improve?"

Any doctor is going to say it is possible. They might qualify [by saying that] there is a very slim chance. As a physician, I know what that means, but I wanted to believe in a chance. The rest of my family felt if there was a possibility, we should keep Dad alive and give him time to recover.

Days passed, maybe a week or two, and he ended up requiring a feeding tube. I know as an oncologist and as someone who deals with people who are very sick that a feeding tube is often one of the last things that is going to happen.

My family decided they wanted to keep him going. He was even on a ventilator for most of this recovery period, and they talked about placing a tracheostomy tube for the ventilator. I was gently advising them to consider not doing those things, but I was overruled by them, and maybe sort of overruled by my own heart and optimism.

The feeding tube led to unexplained bleeding, and he ended up again getting many units of blood. Then the family eventually came around to facing reality and we let him go.

What is interesting about the whole experience to me is that, as much as I felt like I had the expertise to provide guidance and judgment to my family, I found myself wanting to believe, wanting to be optimistic.

Matt found his father was stripped of his identity during his prolonged hospitalization and ICU stay.

Culturally, we do not view death with the dignity and honor it deserves. I think we view death as a failure. There is something dehumanizing about the way ICUs and hospital rooms look. People in the ICU are wearing a ridiculous piece of fabric tied around their necks. They have tubes in their arms and are connected to a machine. Their heart is a beep on a monitor. They have no dignity. We treat them like a science experiment. If that person was in their bedroom and we walked in and they were wearing their finery, or at least their own clothes, and were surrounded by their family, we would treat them differently. People have recognized for a long time that medicine/medical care is not dignified. Do we do that to patients intentionally so that we can do undignified things and feel okay about them? I don't know. As a society, we should honor and prepare for death so that we can die with dignity.

Matt's friendship has helped me navigate the loss of my younger sister, and I believe I've been able to help him weather the impact of losing his father. As I learned in our conversations and discovered again and again through my interviews with other physician colleagues, each of us has experienced painful losses; armor-piercing moments full of doubt, dread, failure, or overwhelming sadness. We tend not to share them with each other, but keep them to ourselves, soldiering on, seeing one more patient, working one more hour, avoiding the quiet moments when grief presents itself.

GUS MAGRINAT

Gustav "Gus" Magrinat is an oncologist with Cone Health's breast cancer program. He came to the United States from Cuba in 1961, attended high school in Saint Louis, and graduated from Harvard University with a degree in English literature. He was a social worker for two years, then pursued a career as a freelance writer until he decided to go to medical school. Two decades after finishing college, Gus graduated from the University of North Carolina School of Medicine, completed his residency in internal medicine, and did a hematology and oncology fellowship at Duke. He has practiced in Greensboro since 1993. Ever-curious, he also earned a master's degree in pastoral studies from Loyola University in 2004.

Gus is slightly built, soft-spoken, calm—always seemingly at peace. He approaches people with curiosity and attention, often with a twinkle in his eye. Never seeming distracted or judgmental, he is completely focused in conversation. He is passionate about his patients; his wife Mary and their son and grandson; social justice; religion and philosophy; and the outdoors.

I knew that Mary Magrinat had breast cancer many years earlier and I wanted to understand what it had been like for Gus and Mary to go through that as a couple, as well as how the experience affected him as an oncologist specializing in breast cancer. When we spoke, Gus had recently lost his father and mother and had to make difficult choices about withdrawing care. How was it that he was always so serene and accepting? I wanted to know how his religious beliefs informed his patient care and his thoughts about dying. I was eager to learn his perspectives and hoped, in the wake of Victoria's death, that some of his calm and acceptance would rub off on me.

After college, Gus spent time as a social worker in Bird S. Coler Hospital, a New York hospital for chronic diseases. This was when he first came face-to-face with disability and death. He was outraged by what he saw: patients were sent there to be housed and to die.

I can remember my reactions, so I understand other people's reactions when they come across death for the first time. Basically, we grow up thinking that we will live forever and everybody else will live forever, and that a few people die, but that is their problem and that is their fault. *I am not going to die.* And then, at some point, you understand that this is happening, that it is real, and that it is going to happen to you someday. When it does, then one's life trajectory changes.

In *A River Runs through It*, Norman Maclean writes about the way a river runs. People think a river runs straight down. And that is not how a river runs. It runs one way until it hits a rock, and then it runs another way until it hits another rock. So, a river hits rocks and changes course. And that really is how life is.

I use this image when I talk to my patients, and they often find that fits their experience. They are not going crazy; it's normal. They have just hit a rock, and they cannot go in the old direction anymore. They have their marriage and their lives and their kids. They have to get back to that, but it is not going to be the same. Nothing is going to be the same. They are heading in this direction now, and eventually they will hit another rock, and then change. And, eventually, they will arrive at the ocean.

This brief experience in social work profoundly affected him, though it was many years before he decided to go to medical school.

I ended up in oncology. Nobody had signed up for the oncology rotation, which was supposed to be depressing, so they put me on that service. I think oncology is the very best of medicine. You have great relationships with the patients. You don't have to convince them to quit smoking or not to eat so many carbohydrates or exercise. They want to become vegans! They are very motivated. They want to learn. You get to meet the family. Everybody is involved. You become part of that. . . . You have these long wonderful relationships that have great intensity. In oncology, the patient-doctor relationship is the best there is in medicine—that's my view!

At the same time, the science is absolutely fascinating. It is basic cell biology, you know. So, great stuff on both sides, and that worked for me. I kind of fell into it by accident, I suppose. But I love what I do.

He believes it is part of his job to help a patient die in the best way he or she can, with the least suffering and the most awareness: "the best forward-looking plans." And when this happens, he tells me, he doesn't feel bad. "I miss them, I like them, I love them, I feel close to them, but if I have been able to help them through the death they have, I feel very positive about that."

Gus observes that many patients want to avoid talking about death and traces this back to cultural priorities. "What our society sells is sex and food and pleasure and youth. It doesn't sell death and suffering and darkness and depression. Sex and food is what's out there, and that's what people consume. Is that healthy? I don't know. I don't know how it is in any other society. This is the one that we live in.

"We need a more practical—a more realistic—understanding of death, because if not, then it gets very expensive and resources are wasted. Our pharmaceutical and healthcare leaders, our political leaders, are clueless."

Families, too, play a major role in coping with an illness.

Most of the time this is straightforward: What can we do to help? What is our role? A special issue has to do with family members who live far away or have been estranged. They feel a need to demonstrate love and concern, and sometimes they do this by challenging the doctor's motivations or recommendations. The best response in my experience is not to become defensive, but to say "I can tell you really love your relative." That is the point they are trying to make. Usually we can move on from there. In most cases, though, family members just need direction. The goal is for the patient to be safe, comfortable, and able to make their own decisions until the end. Most families do a terrific job with that.

After a patient dies I will frequently send a note to the primary caregiver. This is an opportunity to praise the patient for his or her courage or faith or consideration of others, but also to mention the incredible amount of work the family did in the last few months of the patient's life. So many people have a feeling of guilt, thinking they perhaps did not do enough. Most of them have done a truly heroic job. Mentioning their self-sacrifice I think is helpful as they move on to grief and, eventually, comforting memories of the one they lost.

He does not see a great difference when treating cases where there are physicians in the patient's family, other than it "means that I have to be on my toes. These are people who are going to be able to get nuances, so I had better know what I'm talking about. Not just the gross picture but also minute facts. Otherwise, they lose confidence. That's really the only difference. Otherwise, they are just people."

I spoke with Gus about Mary's illness and how it affected them both, though he readily admits it had a far more profound effect on Mary. "By the time she got sick, I was in medical school. I had already experienced death and dying. My concern was to care for her, to make sure that she was okay. I was expecting her not to die. *She* expected that she would die, but I did not expect her to, so I never had the feeling, *Oh my gosh, she is going to die.* It was difficult for both of us. The main thing was we could not have more kids . . . but you know, that's life."

His father and his mother both had advanced dementia when they died.

I did not prolong their dying process. I did not interrupt it. My father died from a urinary tract infection that we did not treat, and he became septic and died. He probably had prostate cancer, but we never worked it up. He had terrible dementia. He was in a nursing home. His second wife, whom I love, couldn't really take care of him anymore. There was no life there. I mean, when I visited him, he thought I was a thief. It was dreadful.

When they called to ask my advice, I said absolutely not, do not give him an antibiotic. In the end, they gave him some, but it was too late. He died in the nursing home within two days. He was unconscious [that entire time].

My mom stopped eating. She was also totally demented. When you put a spoon in her mouth, she bit it. She stopped eating, so she died of dehydration. I could have given her IV fluids or done some intervention, but what would that have accomplished?

I don't think either of them suffered. But the emotional part is separate from that. The actual, physical process of dying is not a big deal. The emotional part is a huge deal.

His parents' deaths also increased Gus's sensitivity to the suffering of his patients and of their families by adding a personal experience of their circumstances. "You have a better idea of what they are going through. You understand why they are crying nine months later and longer than that."

I asked him if he thought he would make different choices for himself as a patient with a terminal illness than he would recommend to others.

It's very hard to know. I know that if I was suddenly diagnosed with pancreatic cancer, I would feel very vulnerable. I wouldn't feel neutral about it. It would be like getting hit in the gut with a baseball bat.

I realize that it would be a major issue no matter how much I've prepared myself, but then, would I take some Gemzar even though it really doesn't work well? Probably, I would. I would give it a shot. I don't think I would be very interested in things that prolong life at terrific cost in quality of life. I think it would be a reasonably quick transition, so I just would want to be comfortable.

Let's make sure I'm comfortable. If the drugs that make me comfortable hasten my death, then that's okay, too. I think I would be kind of like my patients, but a little less hopeful because I know the odds. I know the statistics in a different way than my patients do. I've provided the statistics to each of them, but I have seen the numbers play out more often than they have. So, I feel a difference.

There's always hope. So the motto of hospice is: No one should die alone. No one should die in pain, and no one should die without hope. Yes, there's always hope. The day before you die, there's hope . . . But it is a different experience when you are the one who is in the process of dying.

Gus has clear ideas of how we should improve the delivery of medical care in the US but says that under the present system, his obligation is to his patient rather than to ration resources for the greater economic good.

I'm prescribing drugs that cost $3,000 to $10,000 a month that my patients have to buy at the pharmacy. I think we need a system of rational rationing.

Then everybody will get what they need up to a point. Beyond that point, they won't. But do you want to run on that platform?

If I feel treatment is futile, I say, "You know, I really think it's futile. You could try it, but I wouldn't. It's got side effects. It's not going to make you live longer. You're going to die just the same. It may make things worse, and in the meanwhile, you're not doing what you really need to be doing." I don't feel that I'm obligated to prescribe something just because it is out there on the market.

I'm very clear that my job is to treat the patient, not to solve the general problem of medicine in the United States. Whatever I can do that will help this patient, even if it is incredibly expensive, which it is, I will do. The cost of cancer drugs is ridiculous.

A cost of $50,000 to $150,000 a year is not uncommon for cancer treatment, and radiation alone is $50,000 or more for six weeks. I mean, it's ridiculous. The point is, if it will help my patient, my society says it's okay, so that is what I do.

Gus's religious background has strongly informed his medical practice. Brought up a Catholic, he left the church in his teens, became a conscientious objector during the Vietnam War, and later joined a Quaker Meeting in Greensboro, attending for many years. That was where Mary and he met, and they were married in care of that Meeting. When Mary's brother Eddie died at age twenty-four in a car accident, they returned to the Catholic church, where she felt more at home. "By then Vatican II was transforming Catholicism. My feeling now is that there is no perfect church. Catholicism is as good as any of the major traditions, and it has a very sane understanding of science. It's the one I know best—I completed a master's in pastoral studies through Loyola— but I could be Lutheran or Methodist or Jewish. I don't know enough about Islam. I do think there are truths, like the value of every human life, that are not scientific or political. That's the great value of religion."

Victoria showed a growing sense of gratitude as her illness progressed, and I asked Gus if he had witnessed something similar—and if he himself approaches the idea of death this way, as he seems to exude gratitude and calm. He has thought a lot about this and about how his religious views intersect with his sense of his own mortality.

How do people react to death in general? And their own death? I think most people do not want to face death, so they don't.

In the Judeo-Christian religions, although apparently there will be no sex in heaven, people are going to feel really good, and everybody is going to be there. We have this hope that everything is going to be wonderful. A lot of people jump from "Oh, I just got lung cancer stage IV" to "*Boom!* I am going to be in a great banquet with all my friends and family. It is going to be terrific." But there is a process to go through to get there.

Most people don't face the reality of death. Those who do and [who] live long enough to experience the suffering that is involved react in different ways.

I am amazed at how many people make a positive out of it. They hate to be dependent on others, but they accept it like it's a job. They conclude, "It is my job to suffer, to be a patient, someone others must take care of."

They become grateful for little things. I do not know exactly how it works, but it is not that uncommon. It is a wonderful response. They do not respond like victims, although some people do think of themselves as victims and feel angry and can't accept what's happened.

While I don't share Gus's religious views of an eternal life (nor did my sister), he doesn't impose his beliefs on others but uses them as an internal guide. He is sincerely interested in his patients' perspectives and works within their belief systems in terms of providing explanations of therapies, expectations of an illness, or transitioning to hospice care. Driven by empathy, he bases his discussions with patients on his understanding of their desire for information rather than on his need to explain things to them. Patient viewpoints are important to him, and always welcome, though he does express limits: when patients push homeopathic or alternative therapies, he redirects them toward biologically based therapies. He doesn't refuse to allow alternatives but makes clear that he has no knowledge of their efficacy and that they don't play a role in the standard treatments for cancer at this time.

After speaking with Gus, I realized that as a physician I am also comfortable tailoring explanations to patients based on my understanding of their desire for detail and honesty. Gus has developed perspective on his patients' illnesses and the limits of his ability to cure them. He is comfortable working from what he perceives to be their need for explanations, going to great lengths to make sure patient and doctor understand each other. I also saw, in our conversation, that the essential distance dissolves when someone close is mortally ill. And, just as Gus did, I learned that emotional complications arise when we attempt to simultaneously play the roles of doctor and family member.

STACY WENTWORTH

Stacy Wentworth grew up in a small farming town in Illinois. The daughter of a fourth-generation farmer and a teacher, she completed college and medical school at Wake Forest University and worked as a radiation oncologist in Greensboro, North Carolina, where she was also the medical director of Survivorship and Wellness through the Cone Health Cancer Center. While working at Cone, she married Todd, the love of her life, and they live in the country with a menagerie of animals including three rescue dogs, a white cat, two fainting goats, and a large black horse named Sebastian.

She and I worked together during the initial phase of building our brain tumor program. At one point, before Victoria became ill, Stacy told me the story of her aunt Diane, a nurse who went on to become the vice president of a small community hospital in Decatur, Illinois, and then developed a malignant brain tumor.

Aunt Diane was the matriarch of Stacy's family. The oldest sister, she was in charge of her parents' healthcare. "In her retirement, she went from being a busy and effective administrator to running a DJ business and planning events, dances, weddings, and bar mitzvahs. She began training West Highland terriers, traveling all over the United States for dog agility competitions. She ended up a grand champion of dog agility at the Westminster level."

Diane's husband, Paul, "was very much the yin to her yang." In August 2011, on the road in California, she had spells of light-headedness and noticed a strong acidic smell. She was concerned because her Uncle Merle had died of a glioblastoma ten years before and those were the same symptoms he had described.

On her father's side, Stacy's family are all robust farmers, who die either of brain tumors or of old age, at one hundred. Diane was concerned enough that when she returned home, she had a CT scan of her head and an EEG, which came back normal. She then had an MRI, which was *not* normal; it showed a large enhancing lesion in her left temporal lobe, spreading into the right side of the brain across the corpus callosum with a lot of edema. Diane and Paul knew what it was, and Stacy did, too: primary brain tumor.

Diane was totally healthy. Paul had some heart issues a year prior, so they had both been losing weight and had radically changed their diet. She sent Stacy an email describing what she felt was a seizure.

New-onset seizures in an adult are rare, I told her, and suggested that she was probably tired from being on the road so long. Looking back, I realize that was my first denial that something was very wrong.

She knew exactly what she had, and I knew. I trained at Wake Forest with Ed Shaw, who is one of the world's experts in brain tumors; 75 percent of the patients I saw as a resident had brain tumors. I was familiar with this story. My training program, also known as "Ed Shaw's house," had prepared me well in the realm of brain tumors and how to manage them.

My aunt was sixty—in her prime. She had become burdened by her responsibilities as an administrator at the hospital, and you could see the weight lift off her shoulders when she retired. After her tests, she consulted her local physicians, one a neurosurgeon and one a medical oncologist. Ironically, Diane had hired them both during her tenure as VP. This was central Illinois, not exactly a brain tumor center of excellence and not anywhere close to an academic and research center.

Still, Diane had a lot of confidence in these two doctors. I work at a community center as well, and I know that I take excellent care of my brain tumor patients. Yet my first impulse was to get her to a large renowned academic hospital. *I've got to get her to Wake Forest, to the people I know,* was my thinking. But this would also be ripping her away from the nursing staff in Decatur who loved her, and from the doctors, whom she trusted, as well as from friends and family and the dog community. That was really hard for me.

I spoke with her neurosurgeon and her medical oncologist on the phone. We knew that she was going to have a subtotal resection, scheduled for October. She sent me an email; the subject read, "Day of surgery." Beneath it, her message was succinct and clear. "Surgery will be at 7:30 on October 1. I am to be at the hospital at 6 a.m., first one on the schedule, which is exactly the way I want it. Love, Diane."

Diane recovered well following her surgery and began chemotherapy and radiation therapy. She did well for the first three weeks. Normally, Stacy would see her patients on a weekly basis. But with Diane, "I was in the weeds. I monitored her symptoms every day. What might the nausea mean? What were the implications of her constipation, her diarrhea, her lab values? I was not interpreting these things as a doctor; I could not get enough perspective on her situation. There were too many data points. It suddenly dawned on me that I didn't know what my patients go through on a daily basis."

On her second follow-up scan Diane had progression of disease and she was experiencing more symptoms clinically. Still, Stacy clung to the idea that this represented "pseudoprogression," an inflammatory reaction, rather than an aggressively growing cancer that was not responding to treatment. Her aunt's scan had a lot of swelling and a lot of contrast enhancement (which indicates an aggressive tumor).

At this point, Stacy intervened in Diane's care and convinced her doctors to continue the temozolamide and to add bevacizumab in order to cut down on blood supply to the tumor, suggesting it was pseudoprogression. She sent them journal articles "to educate them." At Wake Forest, this had been a well-understood phenomenon: just because a subsequent scan looked worse, it didn't necessarily mean a recurrence of the disease. But, two months later, a third scan showed that the tumor was growing and that Stacy had been wrong.

Stacy felt Diane gave up after the second scan. Despite changing chemotherapy, her aunt became an invalid. In January 2012, a year and a half before she died, she went on high doses of dexamethasone (a steroid to reduce swelling in her brain) and never came off of it. Diane's doctors had started bevacizumab, per Stacy's recommendations, but it did no good. Stacy saw a big change in Diane's personality during this period.

She wouldn't open up to anyone. I think she and Paul had discussions about dying and what was going on, but she would not talk to the family about it. Sometimes we felt she was not trying, not fighting. She wouldn't talk, she wouldn't eat, she wouldn't walk. She would come to family events, and after maybe ten or fifteen minutes she would have Paul take her home.

My aunt knew what she was facing from the very beginning. The wind was taken out of her sails after that first post-treatment MRI. She knew what it meant but was willing to play along until the second scan. She was otherwise healthy, but she gave up, and then the disease started to ravage her. I looked through the emails that she started sending me and noticed she was confusing her words and losing her sentence structure. She was misspelling words, which was so unlike her. Clearly, the tumor was impairing her ability to write and communicate.

Our family struggled because we wanted to push her; we wanted her to step up and be in charge and be "strong" like she always had been. My uncle, however, always supported her wishes. At one point, Diane wondered whether she should come to North Carolina for a second opinion. Her family was urging her to go, but I knew that with irinotecan and bevacizumab, there is only a 10 to 15 percent response rate. I knew there was nothing else out there, really.

The deck was stacked against her, but there was this "swing for the fences" mentality. Why wasn't she mad? Why wasn't she fighting? In retrospect, [I see that] she knew this was a fight she could not win.

Diane understood that balance between the benefits of a larger state-of-the-art health center and entrusting her care to her local team. The fact that she saw something in her community doctors meant something to her niece.

At the end of the day, my aunt put her trust in her own physicians, whom she knew. After all, it was she who had hired them in the first place. And she was right. That was hard to swallow, because I think I was wrong about the pseudoprogression. Her tumor really was getting worse, and her poor test results were not just a reaction to the treatment. I told her to stick with her local health team.

This was Stacy's first experience as a medical professional facing a serious family illness. "The competency of a physician takes on a new perspective when they are taking care of a family member," she says.

> During the last month, they brought in hospice and she died at home, as was her wish. She had always wanted to be at her twin grandsons' birthdays in California, so that year, she was able to throw a fourth-birthday party for them at her house in Illinois.
>
> She was able to celebrate her father's ninetieth birthday at their house. I was just starting a busy practice here in Greensboro and was not able to go back and forth easily. I kept in touch by email and tried to advise her son when the best time to go home might be. She died in June, when everyone in our Greensboro practice happened to be on vacation, so I couldn't go back for the funeral, which I think killed my father more than anything. The only time I could leave work was two weeks later. That was very difficult, but there was no one else to cover my patients. I couldn't leave, and I also knew Diane would have understood and given me her blessing, but I underestimated how important it was to go home to support my father and the rest of my family.

Two months later, Stacy's grandfather died of a massive stroke. He came in from mowing the yard to have lunch and collapsed—her grandmother found him slumped over in his chair. Stacy got a call while she and her husband were on vacation. In their nineties, her grandparents lived independently on their farm and refused to move into town, but they took care of each other remarkably well.

Stacy talked to the emergency room physician from their rented beach house. He wanted to transfer her grandfather to Peoria, where they could intervene and operate. The ER physician was pressuring her grandmother because she'd told him, "No. Absolutely not. He would not want that."

Her grandfather's other brother, John, had died two years before of a massive stroke at the age of ninety-five. He had been in nursing facilities, uncommunicative, and her grandparents saw that and discussed their wishes between themselves, deciding they didn't want heroic interventions.

That day, Stacy's grandfather spoke to her cousin Laura in the emergency room, wanting to know how her day at school had been, and then he never spoke or interacted with anyone again. He was transferred to Comfort Care on the same hall where Diane had been, which was hard for the whole family to revisit. Yet they had a good experience because the nurses and staff had known Diane well. Stacy felt her grandfather received excellent care.

Her grandmother told her that he was unresponsive, so there wasn't a rush to come home. "He is very comfortable. There are a million people here with him. We will tell you when the funeral is." From a physician's standpoint, Stacy knew that her grandfather was not going to wake up.

> My dad called: "No one is doing anything. I feel like he should be transferred; why aren't we doing anything?" I had been all-hands-on-deck with Diane, but now it felt like it was time to drop the mike and walk off the stage. Letting my grandfather die peacefully was the best you could hope for in a ninety-year-old.
>
> I, too, was struggling with how differently we approach each critical situation in caregiving. There is an old adage: "Farmers can only die in the summer because the crops are already planted and there is no harvest." At the funeral, everyone smiled at my grandfather's timing. Even though he hadn't been on a tractor in years, all his neighbors and farmer friends came to his funeral.

These experiences have changed Stacy's approach to her own patients. She told me she was now more aware of the side effects of what we choose or recommend at home on a day-to-day basis. She talks to patients in more detail than she used to about the pros and cons of the treatment decisions we make.

A case in point was a patient she had been referred who had a cervical spine metastasis. It was a new diagnosis of metastatic cancer and she had a compression fracture, but it wasn't causing symptoms, yet. The patient was an older woman who lived alone. Stacy was worried she would develop horrible esophagitis/pharyngitis, become dehydrated, contract a UTI, sepsis, or pneumonia, so she spent a lot of time with her going over the implications of treatment.

The patient and her daughter elected to go forth with the radiation, but Stacy has become more aware that the majority of care goes on outside of the exam room. She now considers not just solving the problem in front of her, but also how the treatment will affect those who will live with the day-to-day consequences; she talks with patients earlier and more often about hospice and about what we can offer. Stacy also attempts to set realistic goals for patients and their families. She notes that none of her aunt's doctors spoke with Diane at the beginning and said, "This is most likely a terminal illness. You have at most a year to live if we do X, Y, and Z. If we don't do X, Y, and Z, you have a couple of months. What can we, as consultants, do to help you in that limited time frame?" She wants to use those consultants' skills to help patients make informed decisions about their care.

> I think we need to practice both sets of skills, the one that treats the patients and the other that counsels them. Or we need to defer to social workers and palliative consults when we are not comfortable doing the counseling ourselves.
>
> I think what is important is where the light gets in. I gave my first eulogy for one of my patients, Treva. I didn't do very well and ended up crying through most of it. She was one of the very few patients; she still gets me. I knew her and her kids very well. They would come to my office, dig through my desk, and get candy out of my drawers. Todd and I went to several of their soccer games; we bought her a T-shirt in Las Vegas. Treva was larger than life. She made us all believe that she could beat the odds. She had an incredible attitude and strong faith. I paid for her burial. I think occasionally some patients have to put a chink in your armor to keep you honest with yourself and with your feelings.
>
> I think occasionally I have to let patients in to make sure that I am not getting too far away from the reasons I chose this path in the first place. Do I risk burning out earlier? Is it unhealthy for me? Is it harder on my family? Is it harder on my husband? Maybe, but some patients, like Treva, refuse to see my armor.

Stacy is not sure how useful all the treatments we provide for patients are. People want to go down swinging and are reluctant to opt for no treatment. A lot of women with metastatic breast cancer agree to radiation after mastectomy to prevent local recurrence even though distant organ metastases, such as to the liver, are more likely to kill them than a local recurrence. In young women with breast cancer, patients want to actively treat the cancer, in the hope that it won't come back. "Their expressions say, *You just want me to do nothing right now?*"

> The way I have started to approach my patients whom I consider to have low cure rates is to say, "I have to tell you this. Imagine there are a hundred people like you in a room, but only ten of them (or whatever the statistical data shows) are going to be alive at the end of one, two, three years. Whether you are one of those ten or whether you are not, we don't know. We are treating you as if you will be, but more likely than not, you won't be. I am not going to beat you over the head with this, but the odds are not in your favor, and I hope that someday you come back five years from now and say, 'Wentworth didn't know what she was talking about. She told me I was going to die, and here I am watching the Masters.'"
>
> We need to have that conversation because there may be things you need to do, people you need to talk to, wrongs you need to make right, in that time frame. Dr. Richard McQuellon, another mentor from Wake Forest, calls it "living in mortal time," which is the title of his book. It's his term to describe how cancer patients live with illness, and maybe the same is true for those with other diseases as well. The aim is to have a sense when your life will end, and that is a difficult burden to bear. As a sentient being, to know the time of your impending death makes it almost impossible to live. For oncology patients, they have a hard time wrapping their minds around this. The rest of the world is churning along, unaware, and my patients are counting every day, every minute. I have to give them that information because I think it is unfair to hide behind that curtain.
>
> As Americans, we don't talk about death. We put death away, in nursing homes and skilled nursing facilities. I certainly feel ill-equipped when it comes to [having] these conversations.

Stacy is a supporter of living wills but feels they don't go far enough. Rather than the signed document, "it's the conversations leading up to [the living will] that are more significant." She wishes we would offer classes or discussions about death, rather than a six-page booklet that the nurses are now required to have patients at the Cancer Center sign.

She says she came home from her first rotation in medical school in the pediatric ICU and made her family sign DNR orders. She told her parents she did not want to have to intubate them, and she did not want to let them end up in a nursing home. This caused her parents to have a discussion and "it added clarity, especially for my brother, who is a very optimistic person. I hope that in twenty or thirty years, or whenever they die, he remembers that."

I asked her if she would do things differently as a practitioner and if she had ideas she would like to incorporate into her practice.

> I think medical training should occur in two steps. You should have to go back for training after being in practice for five years, at least, in radiation oncology . . . in radiation oncology you're trying to drink from a fire hose just to get the information to treat cancer correctly. The subtleties of interpreting the clinical trials and studies, learning the techniques, the energy, and the physics, and [doing] symptom management—it is overwhelming.
>
> I had one of the best teachers in the world, but as a resident, I felt, *I have so much to do right now that I can't possibly absorb the conversation Dr. Shaw is having with his patient.* Looking back, [I see] what a travesty that was. I would love to go back and be less problem-focused during the training. There was so much emphasis on getting the information as fast as you could, dealing with the patients efficiently, [and then] moving on, because there was always somebody else [who] needed you.
>
> Doctors tend to operate at burnout level. Nobody taught us about work–life balance in residency. We were taught to take care of patients but not ourselves. No one asked me about my mental health.
>
> Doctors have to find a safe place to talk about all they deal with at work. Not your poor spouse—you have to find somewhere to put your failures. Hopefully, the culture is changing; maybe these ideas are being introduced in medical schools today.

Stacy has been grappling with some of the same issues with which I have been struggling. That she is providing radiation to patients, rather than surgery, does not lessen the tremendous sense of responsibility she feels toward her patients. She worries about how she counsels them and has come to see that the impacts of treatments extend far beyond office visits. She learned, through her aunt Diane's illness and death, the limits of her power to intervene and how hope for a better outcome caused her to distort data and interfere, rather than help.

Her stories also helped me see the limited influence that greater understanding provided her aunt in impacting the outcome of her illness. Even with a keen understanding of the facts, Diane was not able to appreciably alter the course of her brain cancer. I had felt, through Victoria's illness, that greater understanding of the facts surrounding her leukemia would have helped her, but after conversations with Stacy I began to wonder how much of a difference this would have made and realized that my uneasiness was a reflection of my own frustration with my inability to alter the facts or to help my sister.

SEAN FISCHER

About ten months after Victoria's death, I flew back to California to visit Pat and my nephews. Sean Fischer, my sister's hematologist-oncologist at Saint John's Medical Center, graciously agreed to meet with me.

I was eager to talk with Dr. Fischer and learn how it had been for him to care for Victoria. I wondered if he had found communication with her a challenge, what his relationship with her had been like, and how he managed the grief of losing a patient. Many doctors would refuse to meet with a deceased patient's family members. They would choose to avoid a potentially angry confrontation with grieving family, especially if there was the perception of wrong, in which case they would be afraid to do so (or would have been advised by their attorney not to meet). Often, they might wish to avoid violating the patient's confidentiality and refuse on that basis. Indeed, I had approached both Drs. Fischer and O'Donnell, but gave up trying to reach Dr. O'Donnell after many unanswered phone calls and emails explaining the nature of my request. I had always had a closer connection with Dr. Fischer than with Dr. O'Donnell, and he immediately understood what I was trying to accomplish with this book.

When I reread the transcript of my conversation with Sean, I discovered that I had spoken far more in this interview than in any of the others. Ostensibly, I had gone to his office to do research for this book but, in reality, the meeting became an experience of comfort and an expression of grief. None of the other interviews were with people who had known my sister. Sean had known her personally; indeed, he had discussed with her exactly the matters that I had hoped to broach, but could not: her perception of her mortality, the reality that her treatment was failing, and the imminence of her death.

Sean had known her from the outset, from before her diagnosis, and knew the day he had received the phone call from the pathologist telling him the bleak cytogenetic test results of her leukemia that she was unlikely to survive this illness. I wanted to understand how he had conveyed those results, how he had managed the tension that I had found so excruciating. I knew that he cared about Victoria—that much had been clear from earlier conversations.

This was the first, and only time, we met, although we had spoken many times before on the telephone and exchanged multiple text messages. I discovered that Sean and I both come from the DC area. He grew up in the Maryland suburbs and attended the University of Maryland, then went to Georgetown University, where he did a hematology-oncology fellowship. He got married, had kids, and moved to Los Angeles in 2005. For the past ten years, he has been in a general hematology-oncology practice with a primary focus on hematologic cancers. He also treats solid tumors, like lung cancer. Sean and his partners help cover each other's practices. He has been focused on bone marrow disease since he came out of training.

I asked what it had been like to take care of Victoria.

> I remember it pretty vividly. She was seeing a naturopath; holistic communities are plentiful out here, as you are probably aware. She was seeing somebody [whom] I know and respect, and somebody who felt this was a little outside of her spectrum. Victoria's case was presented to me as

somebody with anemia. As I reviewed her labs, I noted a couple of subtle abnormalities, to my recollection. She may have had a slightly elevated white blood cell count and some anemia. Based on what I saw, there were a lot of different possibilities, so I recommended that we do a workup to figure out what was going on.

It sounded like she had been on-and-off sick, a subacute illness, almost like viral infections that she had been dealing with on a chronic basis. She had been recovering and then feeling worse again. I remember getting the call from the pathologist [saying] that she exhibited circulating blasts on her peripheral smear and having to call her to say, "This is a bigger problem than we thought."

Then I brought her into the office and went through the likely scenario of acute leukemia and how we typically manage it. I explained how we had to get more information, which would come from a bone marrow biopsy, and that once we knew what general subtype of acute leukemia we were dealing with, we would know how to initiate therapy.

We spoke about what it's like to take care of patients who are focused on naturopathic remedies instead of conventional medical treatments.

It can be a problem. There are certainly patients here and in Los Angeles who feel very strongly about nonpharmacologic intervention for their illness. This was not a problem at all with Victoria because she understood. Victoria and Pat both grasped that this was a potentially life-altering diagnosis and it warranted serious treatment. She asked about other things that I could incorporate into the mix, which I am not utterly opposed to as long as they are deemed safe. She wanted to try to keep that aspect of her philosophy aligned with her general treatment, but it was not an obstacle in her case at all.

A patient I saw earlier today decided he was going to deal with his diagnosis of Hodgkin's lymphoma by changing his diet and taking high doses of antioxidants. Of course, that didn't work, and fortunately we were able to intervene at a point where there was no major impact on his stage and prognosis. But all too often, we will see that somebody comes in and has something very treatable, but by the time they explore other options, they come back with a different scenario down the road where it is not as treatable.

I recounted my impressions of the conversations I had with Sean surrounding Victoria's diagnosis with acute leukemia and the specific subtype of monosomy 7, including the dismal prognosis associated with that diagnosis. We discussed how he shares information with patients and whether he thought Victoria accepted her diagnosis or was in denial.

We talked about my sister's declining platelet count and whether this was an indication of early failure of the transplant. Sean said that Victoria was on an "infinite" number of medications and that drugs, rather than rejection, are typically the first thought for a dropping platelet count. I told him about a conversation with Dr. O'Donnell after Victoria died, in which she said, "Well, we really didn't have anything else to offer her after the transplant failed," because I wondered if this had been a lost opportunity for Victoria to confront her mortality and to have an honest conversation about death. They were starting chemotherapy, light chemo, because they couldn't attack the transplant, but then my sister became septic and died as a result of infection. Neither Victoria nor Dr. O'Donnell were interested in having that direct discussion, so I wondered if they pursued treatments that were unlikely to be helpful partly as a way of avoiding the reality of her situation.

From the time of diagnosis to late stage in the game, I think your sister was smart enough to know that once she relapsed following transplant, there wasn't much anyone could do. She seemed pretty well-informed, so I'm sure she knew how sick she was when she relapsed posttransplant. On the flip side, it may have been that she was holding on to hope. Sometimes doctors will say things like, "We don't have anything right now, but we are expecting to open up a trial," little things that doctors may just kind of throw off out of their heads, not knowing exactly when, or what, or if. Patients really take that to heart.

I think it is good to have a discussion of death and dying, but I think for some people that may not be helpful or constructive, and for a young person, especially with children, it is very different than being an older person who has lived a good life. We get into this debate about whether or not somebody would accept chemotherapy when they have no evidence of cancer, when they are young and they find themselves in this adjuvant treatment predicament. It is amazing, the differences of opinion.

Of course this is LA, and you see people [who] are absolutely opposed to chemotherapy, but there are younger people [who] might say, "If I am going to be around for an extra month to see my kids, then I am going to do anything and everything humanly possible." Then there are older people who say, "If you are telling me that chemotherapy will increase my survival by 10 percent, I wouldn't even think about it. I'm eighty years old." I think for Victoria, that discussion may not have been productive. Perhaps for her family, but not necessarily for her. I don't know.

Victoria was totally blindsided by the events that led to her dying. She had never developed a significant infection after her transplant, so neither she nor Pat had realized what it meant. They were just thinking, *This is kind of standard business.* If that hadn't happened, would she have transitioned toward an acceptance that she was dying? Would they have signed up for clinical trials, or would they have had a conversation? I wanted to know what Sean does in similar situations.

Well, to your first point, I would say they probably didn't recognize the pattern because for whatever reason, we were very lucky when we gave Victoria her induction and her reinduction that we didn't run into febrile neutropenia and sepsis. This is a very common occurrence in transplant patients. So, we got lucky in that respect. I am sure that they went into the infectious risk, but Victoria had not experienced a lot of infections prior to that. I am sure the transplant team told her that with induction chemotherapy as part of transplant and conditioning, we completely wipe out the immune system. That is why, in the transplant setting, everybody is on countless numbers of antimicrobial prophylactic drugs. Infections do happen, even with those drugs.

At City of Hope, transplant patients are on antifungals, antibiotics, and antivirals. There is a whole protocol of prophylactic medications that she was on. What we would typically expect in that kind of scenario, in the event of a posttransplant relapse, is that they might try to reignite the graft with a donor lymphocyte infusion. It is obviously a very individualized scenario, but for a young, fit person, you would hope to tide her over until something better becomes available, understanding all of the nuances of clinical trial enrollment. . . .

There is a huge barrier for patients with potentially terminal disease to get into clinical trials. The requirements are often very strict. . . . In Victoria's situation, my guess is that they were probably trying to keep her transfusion requirements under control, keeping her infection-free until something better came along. . . .

Somebody almost always dies of an infection. That is the most common cause of death in that scenario, for sure.

I asked Sean if he thought that we could do a better job as physicians. What did he think we could improve in terms of dealing with death, in terms of how we talk to and counsel patients?

> I think the profession is starting to change, particularly when it comes to terminal illness, metastatic visceral malignancies, those kinds of things. We are starting to embrace the incorporation of the palliative care component from the time of diagnosis, as opposed to waiting for somebody to get very sick, which I think is a really good thing. This is based on the Dana Farber study that showed an improvement in survival with integration of early palliative care in end-stage lung cancer patients. The survival advantage was a couple of months, which is enough time to get a drug FDA-approved.
>
> As oncologists, we feel like we are good at dealing with symptom management, but we clearly do not have enough time to delve into the psychosocial aspects of things, spending hours talking to patients, or going into patients' homes, which palliative care can do.
>
> I think you have to figure out how to segment your time, and I feel that for me, at least in the way I take care of my patients, getting involved in their lives and understanding them—maybe it's not the nitty-gritty, but understanding the big-picture issues from a psychosocial standpoint—is very important. It helps with my general philosophy about how to manage that patient, how to discuss information with them, how to treat them. It is part of the process. I am not saying I do a good job with it, but I am saying that I try, because I never want to be one of those doctors who walks into a room and says, "Well, this is what you have. This is how we are going to treat it. Come in next week and we will start your chemo." I saw this when I was training and throughout my career, and I just never wanted to practice like that. I would not want that approach for a family member of mine. I try to get to know my patients, and I try to empathize. If you don't do that as an oncologist, you are probably not in the right field.

During Victoria's treatment, Sean was generous with his time, allowing me to call him from North Carolina and ask questions. Had he ever found himself playing the stressful role of medical interface in his own family?

> Not so much with my own family, but with my wife's family—and I try not to get involved. I try to steer everybody in the right direction, because professionally, it is not who you want to be.

I know your position: "We have a doctor in the family, and he can help us translate some of this stuff." First of all, you are a neurosurgeon, so it is hard for you to really weigh in on this. You can go and read about it and get a better understanding than your family would, but blood cancer is not something you deal with on a frequent basis. I thought at least I could give you some insights, speaking colleague to colleague but keeping it simple, just saying, "Well, you know, this is good, or this is bad." Then when your family came to you with questions, you would be prepared to say, "I talked to the doctors, and this is kind of where we are." Just hearing that from a physician carries more weight than going online.

After I learned how tortuous Victoria's treatment was, I took a step back and thought, *I prescribe all these things! I do all these surgeries on people, opening up their spines and skulls.* It was a revelation to see my sister going through being treated. It made me much more aware of the impact of these medications, the drugs, the surgeries.

It does sometimes feel archaic to give very toxic chemicals to patients. I think that chemo certainly gets a bad rap, and there are certain diseases, including AML, where chemotherapy by itself can cure somebody. Take a look at testicular cancer; the therapy has not changed for thirty-plus years because there are really old chemo drugs that work quite well.

I have always felt that transplant is like the holy grail—trying to achieve graft-versus-leukemia without graft-versus-host. It is a really intense, primitive type of therapy, but I think the breakthroughs are happening rather fast now. I think there will be significant changes in the way we practice now and before I retire. I think there will be some major breakthroughs. You really feel for patients where you see something dramatic happen on the clinical end, and yet they're gone. You think, *This patient would have been perfect for this new therapy.*

I mean now with the breakthroughs in immunotherapy, and particularly in lung cancer, you see patients have dramatic responses. You find yourself wishing, *If I had just had a crack at this with this drug, that patient could be here.* That's a hard thing.

One of the things that interested me as Victoria's illness progressed was how she became suffused with gratitude. Despite the difficult situation she was in, she was immensely grateful. Sean also observed this in my sister.

157

Knowing there is a whole army of providers fighting for you, trying to make you better, does humble patients, and Victoria was certainly such a kind person that I'm not surprised.

I remember hearing Pat say that they were inundated with support. . . . I remember them saying, "We're going to take this head-on, and we're going to focus on what we need to do to get better." What a fight she put on. It was pretty amazing.

It's a very sobering profession; you remember the wonderful things about your patients. There was so much to appreciate with your sister.

I appreciated Sean's thoughtfulness and consideration, his skill, and his availability. Throughout Victoria's illness, he answered her questions, replying to texts and phone calls. I saw that he had been gentle and supportive with Victoria, tempering his responses to her questions, not forcing information on her she did not wish to hear. Because of their relationship and the many conversations they had, he did not think she was in denial about her mortality, but all along understood the severity of her leukemia.

Although Sean cared about her greatly, it was essential for him to distance himself from the immediacy of her suffering, to leave work behind, to go home to his wife and children, to run, and to play his music. He had not caused her leukemia and had limited powers to cure it, yet he did his best to ease Victoria's suffering without becoming overwhelmed in the process.

patients speak: the healing garden

Is it true that the wind
streaming especially in fall
through the pines
is saying nothing, nothing at all,

or is it just that I don't yet know the language?
—MARY OLIVER, *WIND IN THE PINES**

To plant a garden is to believe in tomorrow.
—AUDREY HEPBURN

I have shared the perspectives of fellow physicians as they cared for mortally ill patients and family members. But, what of the patients themselves? How has illness shaped them? Victoria's journal gives her a voice that lives beyond her death, but what of other patients whose lives have been irreparably altered, but not ended, by their experiences as patients? I bring you the stories of four patients. Not only were they generously willing to share of themselves, but their stories are inspiring. Each patient has had to reimagine their lives, accommodating to losses forced upon them. In the course of these adjustments, they have reordered priorities and found meaning and purpose.

*From Swan by Mary Oliver, published by Beacon Press, Boston. Copyright © 2010 by Mary Oliver, used herewith by permission of the Charlotte Sheedy Literary Agency, Inc.

The first two are my own patients; they had brain surgery for cancer. In some ways, they couldn't be more different, yet in others, they are surprisingly similar. Irving Lugo is a physician who developed lung cancer that spread to his brain. He continued to care for others while undergoing treatment for lung cancer. William E. Williams is the young man whose brain surgery I described in Chapter Three. He developed leg weakness after his surgery and has had to adjust to this while living with the possibility of his brain tumor recurring. The last two interviews are with Mary Magrinat, a breast cancer survivor, and Sally Pagliai, whose husband died of stomach cancer. They channeled their losses into positive action, creating the Healing Gardens at Cone Health Cancer Center, in an effort to bring the healing presence and rhythms of nature into the sterile hospital environment.

IRVING LUGO

I have spoken with physicians who, like me, witnessed the deaths of family members. I have explored whether it made any difference in their subsequent treatment decisions and, in discussions about prognosis, whether it made a difference if the patient had medical expertise (in the case of Stacy's aunt Diane, it probably did but not as much as I had thought it might). But I had never spoken in depth with a physician who was himself being treated for a mortal illness.

I had the opportunity to do so with Dr. Irving Lugo, a psychiatrist who is being treated for stage IV lung cancer. I got to know him as a patient through our brain tumor program. When he presented with lung cancer, on staging workup, it had already spread to his brain. Matt Manning and I treated these brain metastases with stereotactic radiosurgery. We performed follow-up scans every three months over the course of several years to assess for new tumors, and Irving periodically underwent additional radiosurgery treatments to treat the new areas with focused radiation, at the same time sparing his normal and unaffected surrounding brain.

At one point, we were unable to determine with MRI imaging whether a new enhancing area was a recurrent tumor, for which we would perform additional radiosurgery, or an area of radiation necrosis, the late result of radiation damage from the tumor-killing doses we had previously delivered to a large frontal metastasis—in which case, the worst thing to do would be to deliver additional radiation. Instead, we elected to perform a craniotomy to remove this abnormal area, thereby providing a diagnosis as well as solving the problem altogether by removing this swollen, irritated part of his brain. I performed Irving's brain surgery and it went smoothly. He was nervous about the idea of having his skull opened but did extremely well with the surgery and went home the next day.

Through all these experiences, I grew close enough with Irving to speak with him about my sister's illness and her death, which was occurring contemporaneously with his treatments. I told him that I was trying to come to terms with my grief and, at the same time, wanted to understand the impact that mortal illness in a physician's family has on the physician. In getting to know Irving, I also wanted to know how his illness was informing his decisions and attitudes as a physician. I wanted to know why he had decided to continue working and how he was able to attend to the needs of others while himself coping with stage IV lung cancer.

A native of Puerto Rico, Irving has been practicing psychiatry since 1984. At the time of his lung cancer diagnosis he had recently left his position at Cone Health, where he was on staff, and returned to private practice. When they first came to Greensboro, he and his wife, Lizette, had planned to stay for a few years while Lizette finished her doctorate before returning to Puerto Rico. But she was employed by North Carolina AT&T State University, and before they knew it their daughter had turned twelve, so they established their home in Greensboro. They always felt they would go back, but a few years have become twenty-something. Still, Puerto Rico was always home.

Irving and Lizette used to spend all their free time and vacation money traveling home to Puerto Rico to see their families, but since his illness he has had a greater sense of urgency about doing the things they had once planned for "later," such as traveling to Spain and completing their wills. They went to Madrid, to Seville for Holy Week, and then to visit family in Barcelona. Catholicism is a lifelong part of Irving's culture, and he has raised his son and daughter in the church. He has always been a liberal Catholic, taking the good and ignoring what he does not believe.

Prior to his lung cancer diagnosis, Irving's only health problem had been borderline high blood pressure, for which he was being treated with a beta-blocker. He had always been healthy, never smoked, kept his weight down, watched what he ate. Three years ago, he developed a dry cough that wouldn't go away. Initially, his family doctor thought the blood pressure medicine was the cause but stopping the medication did not help his cough.

Next, his doctor tried bronchodilators, as there was a family history of asthma, and then a course of antibiotics for a presumptive diagnosis of bronchitis. When Irving still didn't improve, his wife pushed for a chest X-ray. This showed an infiltrate, an abnormal patchy pattern, with some nodules, which was initially interpreted as pneumonia, but a second round of antibiotics did not improve things. A second X-ray showed that the infiltrates were still there, and then they did a CT scan. On the scan, they could see enlarged lymph nodes, and Irving was sent to a pulmonologist.

The pulmonologist gave him more medication for the cough and did a PET scan, which is done to assess the metabolic activity of the abnormal region on the CT scan. This demonstrated the lesions had increased radio-tracer uptake, suggesting that they could potentially be cancerous. He said there was a strong possibility that something was wrong, but the word *cancer* was not used. Clearly, it was implied.

I finally had a biopsy. I woke up from the anesthesia, and as I [was] lying there, the surgeon said, "I am sorry to tell you this, but I think you have cancer." Then he walked away.

He told my wife the same thing and left abruptly. This was the first mention of the word *cancer*.

The plan was to give me IV chemo and radiation directly targeting the lesion. I went to the hospital and they measured me for the linear accelerator. I still have the little tattoos that they put on my chest. I was going to have radiation every day, and afterward I would start my first session of cisplatinum. I do not remember the second agent that the oncologist recommended. Initially, I went admitted as an inpatient, the caveat being that they wanted to wait for the biopsy results.

At the time, I was not familiar with the genetics of lung cancer. I was positive for the EGFR [epidermal growth factor receptor] mutation, and because it was stage IV—actually stage IIIB at the time of my diagnosis— Dr. Mohamed, my oncologist, ordered an MRI of my brain. Initially, they found eight lesions. There was one large one and seven small ones.

My cancer was officially designated stage IV. Dr. Mohamed wanted to combine my course of cisplatinum with another toxin, just to be sure.

The treatment of choice here was erlotinib (marketed as Tarceva), but one common side effect is a severe skin rash. When I developed a rash, I was happy, because there is supposed to be a correlation between the rash and the effect on the tumors. Soon, the rash became like a burn, but I didn't complain because I figured the chemotherapy was working. When I saw Mohamed, he gasped: "Oh my God—the rash!" Apparently, it was infected, so I started antibiotics and steroids.

Within the first three months, they repeated the chest X-ray, and the infiltrate was gone. I knew that the cough was getting better. The mediastinum nodes had almost disappeared, and the principal lesion was shrinking. Each time I had a scan, the lesion became smaller and smaller.

Dr. Lugo said that things have been stable for him since he has been under treatment, although the lesion in his chest is still present. While he had hoped for a cure, Dr. Mohamed has helped him understand that this is a chronic illness.

When they diagnosed me, I started looking [at survival statistics] on the internet, and it didn't look good. There were some gruesome numbers, and scenarios where you drown in your own fluid because you cannot breathe. Patients who investigate their odds and are not supported and properly educated in terms of their disease—I can see how they might panic. I certainly did! Metastatic cancer is not my expertise, and as a practicing psychiatrist, I have not kept up with the science of oncology. Mohamed helped me to understand my prognosis. I kept asking him, because your prognosis makes a difference.

The last time I asked him was into my second year of treatment. "Just be grateful," he advised me. "Live day by day. If your body had not responded to erlotinib, you would be dead by now."

That was an enlightening comment on his part. I must learn to accept the fact that my disease is chronic and that the lesion is still there. Some of the lesions were coming back, but I could not afford to stop working.

I had opened my practice, and shortly after that I was diagnosed. My treatment was an enormous financial burden. Blue Cross Blue Shield dropped our reimbursement rate just because they could. What are you going to do, quit accepting BCBS patients? It was not a friendly environment for psychiatry, so I had to close the practice.

Irving received information from the cancer center about of how he could get financial help with the cost of his medication. But he didn't qualify for assistance because he wasn't destitute. "We are in that range of people who do not qualify for aid but are not wealthy enough to maintain treatment without insurance."

The erlotinib was extremely expensive . . . $2,600 a month on top of the medical insurance premium that [my wife and I] were already paying. People assume that doctors are loaded with money, which is not true. I didn't qualify for any of the health benefits. I did not have enough money to maintain these costs long-term, although obviously my family was willing to help. Without my knowing, my sister donated $10,000 to my care.

It came to a point that I was asking Dr. Mohamed to put me on the cheaper treatment because I couldn't afford to continue with the more effective drugs. It was risky since the mutation does not respond to regular treatment. Erlotinib is still the first treatment of choice.

It was providence, I think, that my old position at Cone became available. They knew me, they knew my history. I had worked there for six or seven years before I left and they were really happy for me to come back, even with my diagnosis. As a benefit, I was able to participate in a group insurance; the cost of my medication with coverage dropped to $200 a month.

When you walk in the door as a patient, the first thing that they say is, "We need your copay"—even before "Good morning."

Many patients go through the same thing. Even when you have a reasonable explanation for delaying a payment, the hospital billing office is calling a collection agency. It was an eye-opening experience. Of course, they have books to balance, but they need to remember that these are human beings and that they are in the business of people's health. It has been interesting living on the other side.

Having said this, he feels he has the best team he could ask for given his circumstances. For the last two years, he has been coming to the cancer center for routine scans and checkups. He parks and walks to the hospital and appreciates the convenience and the pretty walkways and gardens.

I wanted to know what it was like for Irving to continue to practice psychiatry full-time while living with the specter of metastatic lung cancer.

Practicing psychiatry for so long, I am pretty self-aware, but those weeks following my diagnosis, when it wasn't clear how well I would respond to treatment, there were some moments.

I remember a particular session involving a patient who wanted to be placed on disability because he had panic attacks when he saw his supervisor. He came to my office and wanted me to write another medical excuse for his work. Unfortunately, I lost it with him because I didn't know the outcome of my treatment, and it was coloring everything for me at that time. I said to him: "Man, you walk through that door, you put one foot in front of the other, and when you feel anxious, you take a deep breath." I told him that I had recently been diagnosed with cancer and that this is what I have to do.

That was the first time and only time I had allowed my own issues to intrude upon my practice. I do not know where it came from. Just because you are a psychiatrist does not mean that you don't need some support and someone to talk to. I told myself, *I am stronger than that, and I always try to respect that professional line.*

The other sensitive subject for me at that time was suicide. I hear the word *suicide* almost every day. People with depression are in misery and they get stuck in their misery, which is tragic. When my patients, who were otherwise healthy, talked about killing themselves, and I wasn't sure I was going to make it or not, that was difficult.

I was seeing patients at that time and was working with this brilliant student from Mexico. She had attempted suicide three times. I decided to tell her about my own precarious health issues. I wasn't sure whether it would be good or bad for her to hear. I felt the need to share my own story with this young woman, not to make her feel guilty, but to open her eyes to the fact that there are many people who really want to live and don't always have the choice. I tried to point out to her that she was not valuing her life. That was the second time that my diagnosis directly impacted my practice.

I asked if he felt time pressure, and if he had limited life left, did he want to spend his remaining days at work?

In the beginning, I was conflicted, because I thought, although we have been in the States all of these years, this is not home for me.

I thought, *Oh my God! I am going to die!* I got on a plane, went to my town in Puerto Rico, and visited the cemetery and my father's grave. If I was going to die, I did not want to die in Greensboro. I started looking into how to get my medical license renewed in Puerto Rico, figuring out how I could join a practice back home. It would not be so hard to do.

My decisions were not necessarily based on work, but [were] more about where I wanted to finish out my life. It isn't about the nature of work itself, because I love what I do. If anything, I think that my practice has kept me going; it provides structure and a sense of purpose. I get up in the morning; I put my energy into helping other people. It helps me keep my issues on the back burner.

If I were told that I was going to die soon, I would go home to be with my people and speak my language. No more speaking English with an accent. I would surround myself with the music, the salsa, all the familiar smells and sounds I knew growing up. I would go to the church. I lived downtown in Puerto Rico, and the church is always open. I would attend Mass and sit on the same bench where my father used to sit, and that [would] be my life. Maybe [I would] work more on my art.

I used to paint, but then you get busy, and all those things are nearly impossible to keep up. So, when death did not come, and I had a better chance of survival, then plan B became not to change anything, just to stay where I am.

This is my life for now. I get up. I take the dog out. I get the paper, which is full of somewhat depressing news most of the time! I make coffee, and I do a lot of meditation. I have a rich prayer life that I've had since I was a little guy. I do a lot of self-sustaining, self-healing work. The support of friends has helped a lot. I was more private, but Lizette insisted on telling people about my illness. I don't know how many prayer circles were praying for me.

When they diagnosed me, I was covering the Student Health Center at A&T as well as my private practice. They heard the cough that didn't go away, and they were worried. I had to tell them what was going on because I didn't know if I would have the stamina to keep doing everything. So, all these women formed a circle around me. They all hugged, and I was in the middle. I was this "stick" coming out. I mean, all that love in there. It makes a difference.

The rosary is an integral part of Catholicism. People were coming by and giving me rosaries, including one from a patient with whom I was very close in my practice. She said to me: "You know there is something going on with you. Tell me about it."

I was in the process of closing down my office, and I [thought] that she deserved to know what was going on. She pulled a string of beads out of her purse. It was the rosary she used at her wedding. "Something told me that I had to bring you these today," she said.

Whatever a person might believe, the spiritual connection is powerful. I think that the more you have accessed that connection, the better. It's a very important part of my life.

Irving has been pleased with his care at the Cancer Center and with his medical team. He feels supported but not because he is a physician. He has found that the staff strikes a healthy balance of providing information and support.

We spoke about how his illness has affected his family.

It is still something we don't talk a lot about. Each time I go to an appointment, my wife texts me, and if I do not answer within five minutes, she thinks something is wrong. But we are good. The exercise of creating our will . . . has put our situation in perspective.

My wife often contemplates her own death. She requested to be cremated, but I told her, "No, I want my full body in Puerto Rico." She balked at the idea, so the compromise is that we are going to have my body preserved for the Mass, and after that they can cremate. In Catholicism, the ashes cannot be scattered. Although every other Catholic will do that, in my tradition, there is a cemetery.

We took care of the graves in Puerto Rico. We purchased flowers for Mother's Day, Father's Day, All Saints' Day. We bought flowers for Christmas. It is a sacred memorial place, and my father's grave is there. As a compromise, my ashes are to be brought to this spot. I asked to have my remains placed in my father's grave, which will be my mother's grave one day, too.

When I became sick, my daughter was in California and read three books on spices for cancer treatments. She flew to North Carolina and insisted on cooking these weird recipes. Initially, green tea was the thing. So, three times a day my wife would knock on my door and bring me green tea. I drank a lot of green tea. It was important for my family to feel useful, like they were doing something.

Everyone has been so kind. My son-in-law, Ben—I love him to death—has been very, very supportive. I was hesitant about involving my mother, because she worries. Interestingly, focusing on me has given her a new lease on life because she wanted me to be well. I think that keeps her going. As long as I'm okay, as long as her kids are fine, she is okay.

Paul, the neurosurgeon in *When Breath Becomes Air*, said he and his wife were going to separate after their residencies and it took his illness for them to get together again. He said he would not wish such a disease on anyone as an impetus for reuniting. There are two sides to this story. There can be some positive, surprising things that come out of illness. Friends whom I have not heard from in forever have been in touch, letting me know that they are praying for me.

I wanted to know if Irving felt that he was making decisions differently as a physician than he might if he were not trained as a doctor.

As a physician, you want to preserve life at whatever cost. And sometimes the cost is pain and suffering and a burden on the family. We have to get to a point where the decision comes from the patient. The physician needs to be a consultant. Often, if the doctor says to do this, then the patient will comply, even as you, the physician, are wondering whether the treatment might be going nowhere.

You are trying to do the best thing for your patient; you are doing everything, and even some more, but eventually you reach a point where you know it's time for an honest conversation.

We say it's not going to happen, but we never know. We need to put certain requests in place. . . . Do I want to be given hydration, nutrition, life support, all these kinds of things? We may have to face these decisions in the future. In my case, I have decided that I do not want any intervention.

There might always be one more medicine that could prolong my life for a couple of months. For me, it's important to be prepared to die and to die with dignity.

You know, my church is against everything that I am saying because in Catholicism you honor life from conception to natural death. Even so, I think people should be given the right to choose whether they want to terminate their life. Prolonging life and suffering or making your family suffer does not preserve your dignity.

Is he in support of assisted suicide, I asked and, if so, how does he reconcile this with his Catholic faith?

In Catholicism, the image of the suffering Christ is very strong, so you align your own suffering with this. I watched *60 Minutes* the other day and they were debating these ideas. They described an elderly couple; the wife [had] become terminally ill and wanted to end her life. Her husband, or partner, was instrumental in getting the law approved in California. They gave her some pills, they took a walk, and then they went to bed. They cuddled and she passed.

The man in the interview described the memory as peaceful. In contrast, another woman was put into an opioid-induced coma and she took ten days to die. The family witnessed her agony for all those ten days.

The point was that if the care provider could have allowed her to die without suffering, isn't that more humane than prolonging the pain? I am pretty clear about my wishes when it gets to that point for me. I would be ready to let go.

We spoke about what advice Irving has for patients who found themselves in situations similar to his own. His focus reflects the kinds of choices that Stacy's aunt Diane had made for herself, to stay local and not uproot to a larger, more famous medical system for care.

Look at your life. What are the changes that you need to make? Focus on each day, on your relationships; find peace in yourself. Prioritize what means the most to you. Materialism is so rampant, and we give so much value to things, money, fame. We don't give value to community and to self-sacrifice, this body.

Be more self-aware; [do] a little meditation and work. It is not a good thing to bury yourself at work, and maybe I did some of that initially. It is important to find balance in your life.

Your relationship with your team of doctors really matters. When I was first diagnosed, my sister, a physician in Texas, said to me: "Just come to Houston." By then, I had met my team of caregivers in Greensboro and felt confident in the treatment they advised. I have heard stories about people who have bad experiences in other places. Feeling comfortable communicating with your doctors and asking questions is paramount.

Irving feels fortunate to have been spared significant side effects from his treatment, such as deafness, which can be the result of some types of chemotherapy.

> If I lost my hearing, how could I practice psychiatry? Not working was never an option, unless they told me I only had six months to a year. Then I would stop. Otherwise, I was going to practice here or in Puerto Rico; I love this too much to walk away.

Approximately one year after this interview, Irving began to experience headaches, tinnitus, vertigo, episodes of light-headedness, "kaleidoscopic" visual events in the right and left lower quadrants, nausea, balance difficulty, and irregular blood pressure. A repeat MRI of the brain did not show significant change, but a lumbar puncture (spinal tap) showed cancer cells in his spinal fluid, a condition known as carcinomatous meningitis. He underwent whole-brain radiation treatments and elected to retire from working as a psychiatrist. As of this writing he continues under treatment for his cancer and further scans have stabilized, as have his symptoms. The staff at the psychiatric hospital threw him a wonderful, emotional, and supportive retirement party. In the aftermath of Hurricane Maria, a Category 5 hurricane that destroyed much of Puerto Rico in September 2017, he has reconsidered his plans to return to his homeland.

It has been a privilege for me to hear Irving Lugo describe his transition from healthy to cancer patient and to witness the decisions he has had to make. His experience exemplifies current *successful* modern cancer care, which converts a previously fatal illness into a chronic condition, punctuated by episodes of treatment. He has tried to maintain normalcy as far as possible, incorporating these treatments into his life as another set of chores, adjusting his expectations as his disease progresses, striving for dignity for himself and his family as a backdrop for his decisions.

WILLIAM E. WILLIAMS

William E. Williams is a slight, bald, soft-spoken man with a winning smile and a hearty laugh. A musician and worship pastor for a large church, he arrived in our local Emergency Room following a generalized seizure at age thirty-eight. I operated on him for a brain tumor at the time Victoria was hospitalized. At first glance, William's head looks normal, but on closer inspection I can see a thin scar and the imprints of the small titanium plates used to reattach his skull to the edges of a surgically created bone flap through his thinned, irradiated scalp. He otherwise bears no outward signs of his struggles with brain cancer. He is now forty-four.

My interview with William was one of the first times I have talked with one of my own patients, years later, about his experience. Other people I'd interviewed were either healthcare providers themselves or had connections to the medical profession. What was it like to navigate the healthcare system without those connections? I wanted William's perspective on being a patient, what it was like to go through brain surgery and overcome a surgical complication, and how he lived with the specter of brain cancer at such a young age.

> I was thirty-eight years old. I had never had any major sickness in my life. So it was a shock. I didn't have any symptoms. No headaches, no blurred vision, nothing. All of a sudden one day, I had a grand mal seizure, and that's how I met you. And it turned out to be a grade 3 glioma. At the time I had no health insurance, so I was able to get on Obamacare and that's how we were able to pay for things.
>
> When I had a seizure, I was actually driving. I had stopped to get gas. I turned the pump on and sat in the driver's seat waiting for it to fill up and that's when it happened. My nephew was with me.

He lost consciousness. His nephew called an ambulance, and when William woke up, he was in the hospital.

I had surgery [in December 2014], and that was to remove the glioma. Chemo, radiation, both started immediately after, like in January or February. And I stayed on chemo for, I think my last chemo treatment was February 2016, a year later. And radiation was like three or four months, so that ended March or April 2015. I did occupational therapy and physical therapy. I made a pretty much full recovery. I still get checkups every six months, MRIs, and so far, so good. And that was six years ago.

At the time of William's surgery, we had to make the decision to take out the whole tumor, and that means being more aggressive. His tumor was growing into and around normal brain (these were the motor control areas of the right side of his body); ensuring removal of the whole tumor meant risking damaging normal brain.

When he woke after surgery, William experienced some paralysis.

I discovered that I could not move parts of my right side—actually, all the right side. My right hand as well. But it was worse on the leg side.

. . . I could walk, but just not well. You go through stages. I remember being in ICU, then they moved me into a regular room. I was using a walker. It just felt like I had a club foot. So, it took me a while to kind of deal with that, and I kept going to therapy and stuff like that so eventually it got back to normal. I exercise and notice that this whole side, my thigh on this side, is shorter, thinner. It took me a while to be able to have that coordination to actually jump or run. I'm right-handed, but I don't use my right side as much as I use my left side. There was numbness and paralysis [in the arm and hand]; it just wasn't as severe as the leg.

Aggressive removal was the best decision we could have made, yet afterward, it felt like failure. I grieved. Victoria's illness was sensitizing me to the continuing effects of my actions on my patients and on their networks of family, friends, and caregivers.

I was preoccupied with worry about my sister at the time, and when William lost the use of his leg I felt both unanticipated sadness and something akin to guilt. He had trusted me. I was the guy who said, *I'm going to take care of you. I'm going to cut your head open. Everything is going to be fine.* If we hadn't taken out as much tumor, it would probably have regrown and the returning tumor would likely have caused him weakness as well. The surgery was the right thing—but the person doing the surgery carries a burden. I had made a commitment to William that he would be fine, and he was not fine. I grieved his loss, but also my own. I couldn't just stuff that grief away and move on to the next patient; I had to feel it.

When we spoke, I asked him what it felt like to have a complication after surgery and then deal with the doctor who did your surgery.

> It's not *what* you said. It's the manner in which you *said* it. I felt like it was going to be like not a big deal.
>
> I couldn't fathom my brain being open. But you assured me that you've done this before and it's going to be fine. So, I went into it with a certain peace. I woke up, didn't know what happened. Didn't feel any pain. I was like, "okay." But then I realized shortly after I woke up that I [didn't] feel anything . . . It's almost like I'm glad that it was that way because I'm a worrier, so if you had told me it could cause paralysis, if you had told me anything like that, I would have been going into surgery with that on my mind.

When he first realized that he couldn't move his leg, he felt panic.

> Because of course I'm thinking about music. And so I'm like, *What does this mean?* That was my first thought. And my dad was there. He was like "Don't worry about it. It's going to be okay." And he started praying.

Was William angry at me? At circumstances?

> Actually Dr. Stern, I was very pleased with you. I'm not just saying that because you're sitting in front of me. When I got out I was singing your praises . . .
>
> I'm grateful. I'm glad I met you. I'm glad that you were my surgeon. And please don't ever feel guilty about anything. You're doing a great job. You're saving lives.

As he worked in physical therapy to regain mobility after surgery, William was also undergoing courses of radiation and chemotherapy.

The worst part about radiation was preparing for radiation. They put this mask on. Oh, man, I cried. And literally it took, the nurses had to give me time. They brought my dad in there and he just consoled me. I just couldn't. I don't know what it was about that mask, and then they ended up giving me one with the face cut out. I'm not claustrophobic; I think that was the moment that the magnitude of what I had already gone through hit me. And then now there was these other steps. It's like, *this isn't over.* I think it's a control thing. Being pinned down by your head and your face and there's holes there that don't move. It was just a lot, a lot to take in. But I got used to it because you have to go every day, like four months.

[Chemotherapy] wasn't too bad. I just had to get used to it because I took the pill, so I was on the pill [Temozolomide] and it made me sick for a while, and it made me very tired. But it wasn't anything like the horror stories I had heard. I was prepared for the worst so it wasn't that bad. I remember being very nauseous but it was more so in the beginning stages and then my body got used to it and so it was fine. Radiation was probably worse than chemo because I felt it. I was experiencing that.

It was about four months before he felt that he was beginning to get back to "normal." Nearly six years on, he still lives with the effects of surgery and treatment. He is on medication, and has regular MRI scans.

The fact that we see no enhancement or return of tumor is very good, but the surgery also meant that William lost the ability to walk with ease; he lost some of his ability to play music. While he continues to work as a musician and worship pastor, the post-surgery paralysis has had an impact.

I've made a lot of recovery, but still not quite. My rhythm is different, and my coordination definitely suffers. . . .

My main instrument is organ. I'm still able to play, just not as well as I've played. My skill level is not, my coordination is not there. . . . Sometimes, if I play for a long time, my hand will lock up. That never happened before. Oh, I forgot that I still have seizure activity. It's nothing like before, but I'm on medications for seizures.

But my church has been gracious, so I still have my job. I just don't play as much. I play when I have to or I want to. But we brought in some other musicians that can handle that and I'm more administrative. I still teach music, I can still sing, so I do those types of things. We just shifted my role a little bit.

William tries not to dwell on his prognosis, which anticipates recurrence of his tumor, but says that of course he thinks about it from time to time. He found his first oncologist—who speculated that with the use of a particular medication he might have seven years to live— unencouraging. So he fired her, and began treatment in Charlotte with Dr. Ashley Love, whom he calls "absolutely amazing." I asked what Dr. Love did differently.

> She gave me hope. Of course, the treatment, well first of all, the first oncologist I had, she recommended a medication that was . . . a dated medication for my situation. So that was the first thing. [Dr. Love] was up on her game. She knew what she was doing. But then on the first day she brought in a testimony. One of the girls that works for her had the same thing I had, and she had been cancer-free for I think like eleven years. So immediately, I had hope. Where this other lady was like, "Well we can try to get you seven years." And [Dr. Love] had a wonderful bedside manner and stuff like that. And I needed that because I was traumatized by the whole experience. After two or three years I moved my oncology back [to Moses Cone in Greensboro].

He is currently seeing my colleague Dr. Vaslow, a brain cancer specialist who reminds him of Dr. Love and makes him feel comfortable.

I asked William how he has managed to deal with his diagnosis, received at a young age, and its aftermath. Not playing in church has been an enormous loss, one he still grieves. He is in counseling to work through issues related to his diagnosis and treatment, as well as with his prior experiences of trauma.

> To be honest, this whole experience was traumatic. And I already have a history of trauma. So I've been seeing a counselor. I've gotten married since then, but my marriage has suffered. You know. . . . It came out of nowhere. And having that grand mal seizure I still remember; I can still see it. I relive that. It was quite traumatic because I could see what was

happening but could not stop it. I had no control over it until I blacked out. I still remember the pain. I had no control over it.

It took me a while, my recovery. I couldn't handle noise. I couldn't handle too much stimulation because it would evoke seizures. I'm a very active musician—loud, moving. . . . My church is a lively church. I would go to church and I would have to sit in the office because I couldn't handle all the activity.

I'm able to drive. I keep that limited, though. I didn't drive for almost two years. It was just too much stimulation. I still consider myself in recovery.

I still play music. I mostly play piano now. It's better in my hands than in my feet. And I can play organ: I just use my left foot and I control my right foot with the pedal. But the grace, I don't know what that's called, but the grace that I used to play with—I feel like I have [lost that]. I don't think I play as good. . . . Other people say they can't hear it, but I know, because I know how it feels. I play for myself. I don't feel good playing in church. It doesn't feel the same.

While much of William's care was covered because of the Affordable Care Act, both he and I are worried about the financial impact a lack of access to healthcare would have had on him and about how this affects other patients. He claimed he had to pay $10, 000 out of pocket for his care. Without this coverage, those out-of-pocket expenses would have been far higher.

At the time I was single and I didn't have much savings because I was just living paycheck to paycheck. So to be honest, I don't know what I would have done. I still have debt. Some of those bills that came I couldn't do anything with them so they went to debt collection agencies. I don't know if you know, but they sell your stuff and they just continue to sell it so it stays on your credit as a bad mark.

For a while I was doing pretty good. There has been twice I had to get [my scans] delayed. One time we did a CT scan because it was cheaper than an MRI because I was paying out of pocket at the time. So, you know, it's been kind of hit-or-miss.

I was blessed because one of my dear friends is in insurance. So when all of this happened, I really kind of checked out, I was scared. I was just like I don't know what was going on. But he was instrumental in getting me signed up for Obamacare. So, navigating that stuff . . . I didn't really have to do it. I had people to do it for me, like, "Here, sign this." So I was blessed in that regard.

[I had] never dealt with the hospital. I didn't even know you could ask for [things]. Just things that they would do for you. I didn't know that you could get free rides and stuff like that. They give you that stuff, but if you are sick and you're trying to focus on your life you're not trying to read. . . . I was super blessed to have a team. I had people that just picked me up and just carried me through that.

Two things that I thought about during my treatment: First, I was so afraid as a grown man and I was imagining—that's why I started donating to St. Jude's—*What is it like for a kid to go through this?* Because you know, I was terrified. So, I thought about that and then the second thing was, *[What] if I didn't have a support system? What if you're single in a new city and you don't really know anybody?* It's really scary.

After our interview, William gave me permission to audit his medical bills to get a better sense of the cost of his care. His total bill was over $155,000. With adjustments, insurance paid a bit less than $80,000. The costs of his surgery and radiation treatments were the same at about $46,000 each. MRI scans were billed at approximately $3,700, while CT scans cost less than half that amount ($1,491), so he saved quite a bit going for CT scans instead of MRIs, although these are far less sensitive evaluations. His out-of-pocket expenses have amounted to about $10,000. Without the Affordable Care Act (or any insurance coverage at all), I am not sure how William would have been able to afford the costs of his care or his ongoing treatment.

I wondered if he ever felt that race was a factor in any aspect of his care.

No, everybody was great.[The] staff is just impeccable. So, no I didn't feel that race was a factor at all.

When I was treating William during the period of Victoria's illness and death, he was aware of what I was going through, and he was always kind to me. When I told him Victoria had died, he hugged me. I remember being struck that someone who was in the midst of his own serious illness and complications found it in himself to reach out to me. I was curious about how he handled his experience of sickness and loss.

> I hold onto my faith, man. My faith has been everything. It's got me through everything in my life, so I became a Christian at a young age. Without God I wouldn't be here. My faith is in His word and so when I read in the Bible where it says "cast your cares upon God, he'll care for you," I try to do that. And somehow it feels better. It gets me through, sometimes it's moment by moment. Sometimes it's day by day, week by week. His word says, "If you keep your mind steady on Him, he'll keep your peace," so when I need peace I just think about the Lord.
>
> . . . It's practical, the things that I believe are true. Sometimes you fail miserably, but you pick yourself back up. There's a scripture for that too, where you may fall seven times but you get back up. So you dust yourself off and try to do better today than you did yesterday.

Whether patients or physicians, we are all struggling with our defended approaches to living. We are learning to open up and feel sadness, feel pain, and to accept these things. In the years since I first treated William, I have struggled my way to the realization that if we open our hearts to those experiences and allow ourselves to feel gratitude, we live richer lives.

> I always considered myself a grateful person, because I've always said thank you and I know that nobody has to do anything for you. But when you are down and you can't help yourself it kicks it up to a whole other level. I remember after the surgery, I had been home a week maybe, and I woke up and every day I was worried about my foot. And I remember that Friday morning when I was able to wiggle my toes, because I hadn't been able to do that.
>
> And I just laid in the bed and cried man, because I felt like okay, I'm gonna be alright. Because the brain surgery is one thing and the paralysis was unexpected so I was like . . . "You know, Lord, forgive me, because I have never taken the time to thank you for the ability to wiggle my toes." The gratefulness makes you see the things that you take for granted.
>
> I used to be really uptight because I was a music pastor and everything, so I want everything [to] be just perfect. And life isn't perfect. And I've kind of chilled out. You know the argument with a friend of mine is like "Why do you care about that? It's really not that serious in the scheme of

things," you know? So that perspective has really been prevalent and I try not to stress about anything so it's not really that serious.

Before, I used to feel like I lived for other people, or I just didn't focus on my own needs. I wasn't taking care of me. And this situation has made me kind of flip that. So it's not that I don't care for others, but I no longer do it at the expense of my own needs.

I told William he seems to have adjusted to his new reality with grace and a degree of acceptance I find inspiring.

I have no regrets, man, because I don't want to. Dr. Vaslow, he's like, "You know, it could come back" and I'm like, "Nah, it's not coming back." You know, that's my faith. I mean, if it does, we will deal with it, but don't be saying that, man, because I believe words have power. So we fight about that. He says that the potential is there because even though you got all the tumor out there's stuff in there that could re-form. Which is why he wants me to keep getting scans every six months.

You know, there is nothing more precious than life itself. It's not like I didn't make any recovery. I made a lot of recovery. I've done very well and most people can't even tell I had anything. It's just that I live with me so I know it. And people who are really close to me, they can tell. I have moments. But my life is spared and it hasn't come back so it's a win-win.

We are often overwhelmed with grief when a family member dies. What can we do in the face of so much loss? How do we pick up the pieces of our lives and start anew? What can we do to give back, to express our gratitude and our remembrance? The stories of Mary Magrinat, herself a breast cancer survivor, and Sally Pagliai and the healing garden they created at the Wesley Long Cancer Center in Greensboro, North Carolina, show how two people answered these questions for themselves and point a way forward through grief to renewal and a positive legacy.

Sally is a landscape artist who believed that creating an accessible garden would heal the earth and become a place of meaning and solace for patients and staff alike. Her father, having developed cancer, was treated at Stanford University. During her visits to California, she and her father spent time wandering the magnificent hospital gardens as he received his treatments. Sally found that the connection with nature made a positive difference to both of them.

She recalled how later, her husband Stefano needed treatment for advanced stomach cancer. He hated being cooped up in the cancer center while he received chemotherapy, which took many hours to infuse. During his lengthy treatment, weeks would go by during which Stefano had little contact with the outside world. Sally felt that the community needed a garden for patients to rest and recover. She believes that only when the earth is healthy can we heal ourselves. She sees a profound connection between patients and nature, a position increasingly supported by scientific literature.

After Stefano died, Sally felt physically ill whenever she went near the Cancer Center. In the process of creating the garden, she discovered that her aversion has begun to dissipate. She can walk into the building, and frequently does, without any feelings of foreboding.

Mary is married to Gus Magrinat, an oncologist whose story appears in the previous chapter. She says that having cancer herself forever changed her. After she sold her health benefits company, Mary was looking for a new challenge and a way to give back to her community. She teamed up with Sally, who had recently lost Stefano. Together, they finalized the design, raised over 1.3 million dollars, obtained the necessary permits, hired construction and landscape crews, and corralled the help of a core of volunteers. Individuals, foundations, and businesses supported the project with donations of funds, goods, and services. It became a labor of love for many people, including many cancer survivors and family members of those touched by cancer.

At Cone Health Cancer Center at Wesley Long Hospital in Greensboro, North Carolina, entering the hospital used to involve trudging from a concrete parking garage to a similarly drab hospital entrance, walking past an abandoned building site that had become a dumping ground for construction debris. The entire property was overgrown with kudzu and other invasive vines and plants, to the extent that when Mary and Sally first toured the hospital grounds, the site was impenetrable. In fact, the first $10,000 grant they received for their project was spent to clear enough brush so they could walk the grounds to get a better sense of the land itself.

As they toured the cancer center with hospital officials, they were told that this abandoned area could never be developed because of the regulations to which wetlands are subject. Undaunted, they asked if Cone Health would donate the nearly two-acre wedge of land for a new healing garden. Cone agreed to allow them to build the garden, but the fundraising would be up to them.

Over the past three years, the land has been reclaimed as a natural area surrounding the Cancer Center, yet it remains a wetland. A thick green wall of towering cypress trees and arbor vitae now blocks the rumbling noise of nearby traffic. Shade trees arch over benches, and Adirondack chairs perch above Buffalo Creek next to an adjoining butterfly garden for families and young children. The garden design is based on a meandering circular pathway with bridges over boggy areas of wetland, past copses of trees, along a small creek and sleeping boulders set in a rolling landscape. Turnouts lead to private areas with seating for rest and reflection. The entire garden is wheelchair accessible.

Sightlines are softened and nonlinear, dominated by organic forms and plantings. The garden is informal, yet carefully conceived and planted. Flower beds spring spontaneously from the earth, full of colorful patches of black-eyed Susans, pink dogwood, arrow arum, berry bushes, swamp milkweed, ferns, hollies, and fuchsia salvia. Tall mule grasses pick up the breeze, bleached to a straw color during the winter months. Songbirds have returned to the garden.

During the day, patients and their families often visit, seeking refuge from the institutional hospital environment. Layers of textures, colors, and knolls create inviting outdoor rooms for community and private solace.

When I asked Mary to tell me about her experience as a patient, I had no idea how raw this still felt to her. More than thirty years have passed since her initial diagnosis and treatment. No longer living under the specter of breast cancer, she has suppressed the powerful memories of her illness, yet they continue to impact her to this day. Her life has been shaped by her cancer and her treatment, and by the illnesses of her brother and of her mother, both of whom died of cancer.

Mary and Sally shared their stories with remarkable clarity. They describe agonizing losses and the renewal that eventually followed. Reclaiming the land and creating a sanctuary for reflection has given their grief an outlet and purpose. The healing garden, with its perennial beauty, offers refuge to those who need it most. This creation has been a powerful step toward healing themselves, healing the land, and bringing us together as a community.

MARY MAGRINAT

> I was thirty-six years old [when I was diagnosed]. Unfortunately, I lost my fertility and the ability to have more children. It was a profound loss, along with cancer. It was very difficult. I was terribly frightened. I had an eight-year old son.

Mary had her first mammogram in November 1985 when she was thirty-five, the age at which a baseline exam was recommended. Everything was fine.

> Five months after my normal mammogram, I am in bed reading a book, and when I turned over, I thought I felt something. So I asked Gus, "Is there something?" Maybe, maybe not. But I was busy and convinced myself it was nothing. This was April. After a few weeks, I went in to see my gynecologist, who reassured me that it was probably nothing, but she

wanted me to have a biopsy to make sure. Somehow, I put it off until early June, after we came back from a week at the beach.

I remember the biopsy. I was awake, and afterward, the surgeon held up the tumor between his gloved fingers. "It's a classic benign adenoma. I think you're fine. We'll send it to pathology and it won't take long." It looked exactly like a small, perfectly round rubber ball. He left the room and didn't come back.

I waited and waited. Gus wasn't with me because he was in medical school in Chapel Hill. The assistant appeared, or perhaps she was a nurse. She told me that I needed to schedule an appointment in the office for the following Monday. I wanted the results right then but she said they had to send the tumor for a second pathologist opinion in Chapel Hill.

So, I went home and I called Gus who asked, "Is everything okay?"

"Well," I answered, "they didn't tell me anything yet, but I have a bad feeling." On Monday, I found myself back with the surgeon at his office. He came in and stood with his back to me, shuffling papers. "You have breast cancer," he said. Later I realized how hard it must have been for him to tell a young mother the bad news.

I asked, "How long do I have to live?" Which is, I know now, a dumb question. He explained that they would have to do some scans . . . a bone scan and other tests. I wanted a definitive prognosis, but he didn't have much information at that point. Later, I discovered that when the Chapel Hill pathologist saw the biopsy, he connected the dots. "My God, she's the wife of one of our medical students."

I ended up having my surgery in Chapel Hill because it made sense to be where Gus was in medical school. We chose a very experienced breast surgeon. I had a mastectomy. I had thirteen lymph nodes removed, and I have had problems with my arm ever since. I don't have swelling, but I do have a partially frozen shoulder. I have worked hard on my mobility, but there are still vulnerable spots. My neck is thicker on one side to compensate. Many years later I had a neck fusion, which I think was related to the breast surgery.

The tumor was atypical medullary, and at that time they had very little data on this condition. I came home, and Gus so wanted it to be over and settled. He wanted us to be able to go on and not to worry, and I couldn't not worry. I made an appointment with a medical oncologist in Greensboro.

"You have a very nasty breast cancer," he explained. "You're very young. If you get breast cancer when you're sixty, you have not as many years for it to come back. You had a mammogram in November and you did not have a palpable breast lump, but in April, you found a lump and you have breast cancer. That indicates it's aggressive, and you are ER/PR-negative, which is also not good."

He told me that I should undergo chemotherapy. The decision was agonizing because chemo was not standard treatment for someone like me at the time and because we were trying to have another child. I would be exposing my body to toxic chemicals. I was told that the chemo would probably poison my fertility.

Scientists were just learning how to treat ER/PR-negative tumors and atypical medullary tumors. My surgeon at Chapel Hill told me not to worry my little head about that. "I am going to take care of you, and you'll be just fine." He was a likeable fatherly-type physician, but that was not what I wanted to hear.

"Well," I said, "I am worried and I have questions."

I read everything I could about breast cancer and called the National Cancer Institute and tried to talk to the director, Dr. Bernie Fisher, but I never got through. My parents wanted me to take chemo. They were remembering my brother's cancer and how he was saved by chemotherapy.

The oncologist in Greensboro ordered more tests on the tumor, and I remember the way I felt when I read the results. The words sent shivers of fear through my body. I had at least a 25 percent chance of recurrence, but probably more like a 40 percent chance. At that time, the average length of life if the cancer recurred was two years. I had an eight-year-old son, Tommy, and I was terrified.

I flew to Miami for a consult with a leading breast cancer researcher. I brought all my medical history and scans with me and was incredibly anxious to get advice about whether to take chemo or not. Instead he just wanted to endlessly talk about enrolling me in a randomized study. I went all that way to come to a decision. I was there about my survival and my fertility. I was furious and crying and honestly didn't know what to do.

"Just take it out of your mind. I'm not joining your study. Period," I told him. Instead, I asked, "What would you do if I were your mother or your sister?

Finally he said, "Take the chemotherapy."

Ultimately, I chose chemo because of the fear of recurrence. I'll never know whether I could have made it without the chemo. I could be here with four kids or I could be dead, but I made the best decision I could.

I took 5FU, Cytoxan, and what the nurses called the Red Devil (Adriamycin). My oncologist decided to do it quickly and intensively to try to mitigate the destructive side effects on my fertility. I took it every week for three months. I ended up skipping a couple of treatments due to very low white cell counts, and it was really rough. Those were terrible months. I was deeply depressed. Each time I took chemo, I felt like I was poisoning my fertility.

Gus came home from medical school in Chapel Hill every single night to be with me and to take care of our son. I continued to work all week—mostly ineffectually—and late Friday afternoons, Gus and I would take a walk to try to decompress me before treatment. When I walked through the sliding glass doors into the hospital, it was terrible. I had anticipatory nausea and all that stuff that cancer patients experience. Eventually they gave me that drug that helps you disconnect from reality. It didn't solve everything and I was still aware of what was going on, but it helped a lot. They still prescribe it today. Ativan.

And then the chemo was finally over. I was 104 pounds at five feet eight with no hair on my body, and I did not recognize myself in the mirror. I looked like a dying person and I felt like a dying person, but it was the poison and so when the chemo stopped, I started to recover. It was like spring with tiny sprouts of hair on my head and my appetite coming back and a little pink in my cheeks. I remember running into someone who said with shock, "You're back." They had certainly thought that I was a goner.

There was a woman right down the street, half a block away, whose child was in Tommy's class at school. She had breast cancer at around the same time as I did. She had such a great attitude all the way to the end, and she was a role model for me. I remember her out in her yard in her swimsuit with her dog about 2 weeks before she died.

Although I came back physically after the chemo, I was haunted by fear of recurrence. I obsessed about it. I also struggled to endure the intense hot flashes of early menopause brought on by the chemo. About two years out, I couldn't stand it anymore. I made an appointment with a therapist because the worry about the breast cancer was driving me crazy. After a few listening sessions, the therapist said, "Okay, you are now as of this moment out of the breast cancer business." Somehow that phrase became my mantra and it helped a lot. Done. Finished. I never forgot what I had experienced, but I was no longer consumed by it.

I wanted to know how having breast cancer had changed Mary.

People often say that getting diagnosed changed their lives for the better—they appreciate everything so much more. There was definitely some of that, but mostly this was a very painful episode thrown into the middle of my life. It was an experience I would much rather have not had. Later I have thought that it was like being stabbed and mortally wounded. Eventually I was able to move on but I never forgot being attacked so violently.

I don't think having breast cancer changed my personality, but of course it changed my life drastically. I would have had a different life with more children.

I learned what it means to be sick and vulnerable and afraid. I tasted some of what it feels like to be dying. This was a gift in a way because it has given me a connection to people who are sick. It helped me when my mother was dying. It has helped me with many friends as they have experienced illness and loss. It has also helped me understand my husband's work [Gus is an oncologist].

I learned just what a lifeline it is to have people reach out when you are sick. Because of the nurses and the doctors and the friends and family who reached out to me while I was sick, I have wanted to give back . . . and have been immensely enriched by the experience of giving back.

I think that my life would have been more innocent.

I asked if she had been pleased with her care and if she thought anything could have been done better.

I feel that I had excellent care. I had the opportunity to carefully consider all my options with lots of input from many sources. Looking back, I would not change any of the decisions that I made.

I am very grateful that we have an outstanding medical community here in Greensboro because I was working full-time and had a young child and my husband was commuting to medical school. It was immensely less stressful to be treated here. I thought the care in Greensboro was excellent and much more personal.

I started getting mad a lot. Later I realized that my anger was really at the cancer. I hated going to the clinic to be poked and prodded looking for a recurrence. In the old days I was always told that I was so healthy. When I had a cath inserted in my chest before chemo began, I remember the surgeon saying, "Let's put it where it will be easy for the nurses to get to." The big fat ugly scar showed with most of my clothes—to this day I hate that scar. That scar is a constant reminder to me and an announcement to others about my breast cancer. One good thing came out of this scar: Gus now tells everyone about the option of placing the port where it is not visible.

Gus listened to me, and as a result, I think he has a better understanding about what his patients are going through. He knows about this in a way that a lot of other doctors don't. Maybe it made Gus more compassionate as an oncologist to have had a wife who went through breast cancer at age thirty-six.

Gus also understands what the husbands are going through. He feels privileged to be with his patients and their spouses during this crucial time of their lives. From the moment I first met him, he has always talked and thought about death a lot. He doesn't see it as something foreign or depressing. He sees it as part of life. That was helpful to me.

I remember when Gus promised to tell our son all about me if I died and to show him pictures of me. This initially seemed callous to me, but then in a deeper way, I understood that he recognized out loud where things stood. He also understood completely when I decided to go to the priest and have last rites because I really felt that I was dying. In retrospect I realize that I was grieving, not just about the cancer, but perhaps even more about the loss of the possibility of more children.

I asked if she had been private about her cancer and discussed her illness only with Gus and her family or if she had been more public about it.

I talked about my cancer nonstop with Gus and my family for the first two years but not so much with the rest of the world. Gus was totally patient, but it was very, very consuming for him and for me. I don't think that was unusual.

I also talked a lot to my sister and to my brother and to a close friend. I joined a small support group, which fell apart before even getting off the ground.

At the time there weren't many support groups and most people didn't talk about cancer. I remember going to a professional lunch wearing a wig—in those days the wigs were awful—and feeling so self-conscious. I was terribly thin, no eyebrows, no eyelashes, my awful wig, and for the most part, nobody said anything. One person asked, "How are you?" and then almost backed away. "I'm kind of terrible, but I'm, you know . . ."

Many people wouldn't look me in the eye. I was young and sick and had a child. Gus was always fine addressing my illness, but many people couldn't face it. When I was first diagnosed, my parents were unable to talk about it. My sister just cried. I reminded her: "I'm not dead yet. Don't cry yet."

One thing that used to drive me crazy was people suggesting this or that reason for my having cancer, like stress or negativity. People wanted a reason for my cancer. They implied maybe my attitude was partly to blame. Strangers would share stories about so-and-so who survived because they had such a good attitude. They would tell me that so-and-so was sick because they were under so much stress. Was I under a lot of stress? Maybe I was. I told myself I had zillions of healthy cells and a few very bad ones. People would counsel me about stress, diet, positivity, and while I knew they were trying to be nice, I didn't find that helpful.

Many years later after Mary sold her business, she decided that instead of retiring, she would try "rewiring." Around that time, a friend introduced the Mary to Sally, a landscape architect who had recently lost her husband to cancer.

Sally told me about how, as she stood in the treatment rooms at the Cancer Center with Stefano, her husband, she had longed for a green place to walk. I told her about how nature soothed me during my time dealing with cancer, about how the trees and the sky would bring me down to earth to a calmness and peace that I craved in the midst of my anxiety. We shared stories, and then she brought up the idea of a healing garden and I was immediately on board.

Our initial thought was to design a little garden out behind the Cancer Center. We both passionately believe that nature promotes healing, and we both wanted to give back.

A few weeks later we met at the back of the hospital and picked out a small lovely spot, but then we noticed a huge empty expanse. We found out that was where the Cancer Center wanted to build a parking garage, but the land was unsuitable for building and it was also a protected wetland. There was no chance of ever building on that site. At that moment our eyes lit up and we saw the opportunity to build a big healing garden. It ended up being nearly two acres.

Gus quietly gets things done. One of his patients' daughters wished to contribute to the cancer center. Gus pointed out his office window at the empty expanse, and they decided to help us explore the idea of a healing garden with a donation of $10,000 to the project. This allowed us to hire an arborist and a crew to do some initial cleanup of the trees and the site so we could see what we were up against. The land seemed impenetrable, a jungle full of poison ivy and choked with invasive plants, but when the stream and the contours of the land were uncovered, we began to see its potential. Sally started sketching, and I began to plan.

The Cancer Center and Wesley Long Hospital agreed to form an exploratory committee, and we met regularly with them. We also met with construction companies and vendors and government officials about permits and wetland rules. It became apparent that this would expand into a huge project, and we were eager to take it on. The committee immediately understood the value for patients and families and staff and gave us tremendous support and encouragement. Our goal was to transform two unused acres into a healing garden, and to raise all the money to build it.

Initially we proposed a budget and promised to stay within the budget. Then we told the committee that we preferred to design the most wonderful garden possible. We wanted to use all the land in the most beautiful and useful way and then we would figure out what it would cost.

We would raise money and build as much of the plan as the donations would fund. It is still a miracle to me that in the end we built everything that we had imagined because the Cancer Center and the community supported us all the way.

SALLY PAGLIAI

Sally Pagliai lost her husband Stefano to stomach cancer when he was forty-five. She is a landscape architect and, as part of the long-term recovery from her loss, she teamed up with Mary Magrinat to create the Healing Gardens at the Cone Health Cancer Center where Stefano was treated. I asked Sally to tell me about Stefano's illness.

Stefano began to complain of stomach problems. We attributed the problems to the fact that he was traveling abroad so much for work. One day, he announced: "Something is wrong." When he went to the doctor, he was diagnosed with metastatic cancer in his liver. His doctors discovered that the source of it was a tumor the size of a pancake on his stomach. He may have been living with that tumor for years.

The news was dire from the onset. The doctors said they might be able to slow it down or arrest the growth for a while or shrink some of the tumor, but they couldn't cure it.

Stefano felt awful and had no energy while he was taking chemo. Once a week he would go into the hospital in the morning and leave completely depleted at the end of the day of treatments. We lived close by so I would run home to manage things and then go right back to Stefano. It was really hard on him. After six months of treatment, we got the good news that the tumors had stabilized. After that first long round, they gave him a little break.

I refused to breathe any life into it. "You are not dying," I insisted. Stefano would answer, "Okay, I am not." During those long months of chemotherapy I thought that if I breathed any air into the idea of his dying, then it would be more likely to happen. Some people beat the odds, and I believed that Stefano was going to be that person. I needed to be the cheerleader not only for Stefano but for our kids, so that is what I did. "Honey, you are going to beat this thing. You are going to live." Stefano would answer, "Okay, I am."

Sally's dismissal of the possibility of death, her refusal to "breathe any life into it," was similar to Victoria's. Sally was determined to reject the idea that her husband was dying, despite clear evidence to the contrary.

Stefano was very close to Patrick, a Buddhist monk, who practices healing that is a form of acupressure/acupuncture. Stefano found comfort and peace through Patrick's treatments. Later I found out that they also had discussions about spirituality, about the power of love, and about what happens to energy after death. These discussions were very important to Stefano.

Despite all the treatments that he had endured, Stefano's cancer came back with a vengeance. Dr. Sherrill started Stefano on chemo again but had to stop it because Stefano was so weak. Stefano and I never faced a big decision to stop treatment because Stefano just could not handle chemo anymore. It ate him up. At this point we brought Stefano home and we involved hospice.

Shortly after this, Stefano's best friend, Billy, from Minnesota and Patrick moved into our home for the last three weeks of Stefano's life to help us take care of him along with the hospice nurses. Taking care of someone as ill as Stefano was tremendously difficult and agonizing work. Our daughter, Bianca, was nineteen and our son, Gianmarco, was fourteen, and the three of us would not have been able to care for Stefano at home without the devotion of friends and the hospice nurses. In the last few weeks Stefano had to receive nutrition through tube feedings and he experienced a lot of pain that we had a very hard time managing. Eventually he stopped being able to talk; he would wince and shudder. He slipped into a coma for about three days before he finally died.

Stefano and I did not talk about dying, and finally he was so sick that we could not talk because he didn't have the energy. Looking back, I regret that because there were so many things that we did not work out together. I don't know if you can be prepared or help your children be prepared when a loved one dies, but Stefano's death came as a very unexpected hard blow to all of us. Looking back, I wish that we had been more open with each other about our fears and about the seriousness of his condition. When he died, I didn't even know what he wanted me to do with his remains.

I wondered how Stefano felt at the time.

Stefano was angry and felt cheated. He had a full and rich life after a difficult childhood. He wanted to continue his exciting career, see his children grow up, be my sweetheart. He wanted to live. He was just forty-five when he died. It just did not make any sense.

If you are lucky enough to go through life with a person you love, you build all these layers that are woven together like a fabric. When Stefano died, it felt as if this fabric was violently ripped. My edges just kept fraying. I kept falling apart because this thing that was holding my life together had been ripped and torn away from me. It took a long time for the children and me to reach some sense of healing, and there will always be a big hole in our hearts.

While Stefano was being treated at Cone Health Cancer Center, I often spent the day with him while he received his chemotherapy. There were times when I desperately wanted to take Stefano outdoors, in nature, but there was no place like that near the hospital. My father, who also died of cancer, was treated at Stanford in Palo Alto, and I remember how comforting it was to walk in the beautiful gardens surrounding the medical center. One of the staff members of the Cancer Center, C.L. Hickerson, stayed in touch after Stefano died and asked if I would be willing to design a healing garden for the Cancer Center. I was interested, but there was impending construction at the hospital in the way, and I also could not yet face returning to the Cancer Center.

A few years later as my life began to piece itself back together, I fell in love with Kyle Jackson whose support and kindness enabled me to move forward. With Kyle, I felt a renewed joy for life and excitement about my career. It was through Kyle that I met Mary Magrinat, with whom I had an immediate rapport. I told Mary about the idea of a healing garden at the Cancer Center, and she was immediately on board. Soon after, Mary and I were walking the grounds next to the Cancer Center, brainstorming. We stood where the Wetland Garden is now and realized, "This is where these gardens need to be." Mary and I shared the vision of a garden that would be a refuge where patients, families, and staff could experience nature.

Sally is now able to go back into the hospital, attending meetings and making presentations in conference rooms. The work has helped her to move past the memory of watching her husband suffer and die.

I feel strongly that it is our responsibility to protect the natural world. When we heal the land, we heal ourselves. The land adjacent to the cancer center was unused and ignored and full of weeds and trash. Reclaiming and nourishing the land inspired and healed me. This was a way for me to transform the memories of Stefano's pain and suffering into something meaningful and beautiful for others traveling a similar path.

When you are sick, you feel that you don't have control over your circumstances. We wanted to give choices in the healing gardens: You can follow this path or choose that one. You can sit in the sun or in the shade. You can be next to water, or you can rest under a tree. You can gather together in open spaces, or you can retreat into a quiet nook by yourself. We wanted the garden to give folks a sense of empowerment.

I know from my experience with Stefano's illness that patients undergoing chemotherapy have heightened sensitivities, so we avoided very strong smelling plants and also anything too jarring or too bold. We wanted a place where patients would feel comfortable and safe.

There were so many hurdles to overcome: the complexity of the site itself, the protected wetland zoning restrictions, hospital requirements, accessibility issues for patients, and the gigantic task of raising the donations to pay for the construction of the gardens. But Mary and I made an indominable team and we were totally committed. With the amazing support of the Cancer Center and the community, close to two acres were transformed into the Healing Gardens over a four-year period.

The garden has proved to be a refuge for hospital employees as well as for patients and their families.

Employees walk through the garden and sit at the tables under the umbrellas eating lunch together. One man told me that he came to the garden

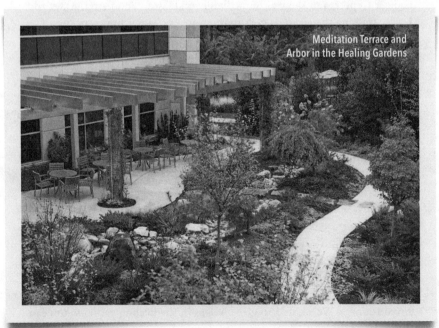

Meditation Terrace and Arbor in the Healing Gardens

Photo and caption courtesy of Mary Magrinat

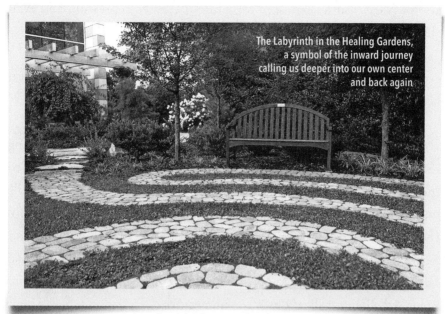

The Labyrinth in the Healing Gardens, a symbol of the inward journey calling us deeper into our own center and back again

Photo and caption courtesy of Mary Magrinat

every day while his wife was hospitalized. Another patient described her routine of always visiting the garden prior to treatment. I see nurses power-walking during their breaks. Parents and children run around and play. Many wonderful folks including patients have become Healing Gardener volunteers who tend the garden. More and more people are enjoying and becoming involved. Witnessing the garden being nurtured and loved has given new meaning to my life, for which I am forever grateful.

Exposure to nature has been shown to reduce stress, decrease pain medication usage, decrease blood pressure, and induce relaxation in patients. According to one study, patients who recover from gallbladder surgery do better with a window view than with a view of a brick wall. Visitors to gardens benefit from tree-lined paths that invite strolling and are accessible to wheelchairs, seating areas that invite conversation, and the proximity of birds, squirrels, and other wildlife. Studies have also shown that stressed hospital employees use the gardens as much as patients and their families do and also derive substantial benefit. Other articles support the importance of walking in and being exposed to nature for our mental and physical health. Exposure to nature decreases depression and even changes brain activity, compared to exposure to urban environments.

Just as I found solace during Victoria's illness while wandering the grounds and gardens at City of Hope, others find peace in hospital healing gardens. Many health systems have begun reintroducing nature into the sterile hospital environment.

Too often, we are cut off from our surroundings, working and living in sterile buildings under artificial lighting. There are no windows to the outside in operating rooms. Day and night become interchangeable under a bright array of halogen lamps. There are no seasons within the constant temperature- and humidity-controlled environment. There have been many days when I emerged to discover that night had fallen or that it had rained and I hadn't even known it. One day, I was surprised when I walked out into a snowstorm.

We have extracted ourselves from the natural world in an effort to create and maintain a controllable environment. Just as we believe we can overcome diseases and our own biology, we have pulled away from the rhythms of nature and the cues that come from the patterns that surround us and of which we are an integral part, often in an effort to deny their importance. There is beauty in these cycles. They are grounding and bring understanding, comfort, and a sense of peace and continuity. By observing them we gain perspective on our place in the world and internalize the reality that, no matter how important, the individual life is a small part of a greater whole. Flowers and plants bloom, die back, but then regrow. We are no different. Death is a natural part of all our lives, and the reintegration of nature into our world reminds us of its importance.

The other day I visited a patient of mine, Ron Evans, an airline pilot newly diagnosed with metastatic lung cancer, which was spreading aggressively. It had invaded his thoracic spine, causing his vertebrae to collapse. Despite two operations to remove the cancer and decompress his spinal cord, he had become paralyzed from the chest down. We were trying to control his disease, but he and his family now recognized that in the end, it was going to take his life. His main concern had become relief from wracking pain.

I was afraid to see him, fearful that Ron and his family would blame me for his loss of function, angry that I had been unable to stave off his illness, although in reality I knew we had done everything possible to preserve, or restore, his function and independence. This feeling of failure was my problem, not his. I was feeling the weight of self-doubt that always comes with complications and poor outcomes as I entered his hospital room.

To my surprise, Ron, and his wife, family, and friends, gathered around Ron's hospital bed, greeted me warmly. They were glad to see me and bore me no ill will. Ron was grateful for all I had done and tried to do for him and was thankful that I had come to spend time with him. It was enough that I cared about him, that he was not alone. His only request was for better relief of his pain. I called my anesthesiologist partner, Paul Harkins, for advice about stronger medications if the increased dosing of sustained-release morphine proved insufficient, and consulted with the palliative care specialists, who could also help with this. Ron was still hopeful that he could be out of pain. He knew he would never walk again. He knew his cancer was not curable and that he was likely to die soon. He and his family were coming to terms with this and expressed gratitude for the care and guidance we were providing.

After my visit, I walked out of the hospital and made my way toward the healing garden. As I followed the steps down, I read the plaques set into the stone wall, the names etched into opaque aqua glass, commemorating those who had died and were remembered, including my sister Victoria Stern Whelan. I passed the trees planted in her and other patients' honor. I stopped, felt the sun on my face, took a deep breath, and listened to the birds singing as they cavorted in puddles on this beautiful spring day.

I walked the pathway, admiring the installations, the boulder field, the marsh grasses, the budding trees, and the colorful flowers. Sitting down on a bench overlooking the garden, I tried to take it all in. Here was a place of peace and comfort, a place where healing could begin. I thought of my sister and took another deep breath and cried.

part
four

CHAPTER TEN

from emotional armor to emotional agility

Empathy is the gateway to the emotional experience of others. How much it nourishes or depletes us depends on the gate swinging back to replenish us through self-empathy and self-compassion. —HELEN RIESS, MD

The year before Victoria became ill and died, my colleague Matt Manning's father developed metastatic kidney cancer and died after a long illness (this was discussed in detail in Chapter Eight). During this time, his father had a devastating stroke. I spoke with Matt on multiple occasions about his father's condition and acted as Matt's interpreter with the neurosurgeon, whom he found arrogant and distant. In our conversations, I also tried to explain the impact of the stroke, as well as Mr. Manning's long-term prognosis from extensive damage to the dominant hemisphere of his brain.

Matt was a valuable resource for me when Victoria became ill. We talked at length about leukemia, of which I knew little. He was able to coach me through her bone marrow transplant, including the pretransplant conditioning, with its near-lethal doses of radiation. He remained a supportive and knowledgeable friend when Victoria relapsed and when she died, I turned to him for solace. I also wanted to understand how he was able to bounce back from his father's death and how he managed to keep functioning as a kind and empathetic doctor without crumbling.

Two months after my sister's death, Matt and I talked late into a fall evening, sitting on the porch at my home and looking out onto Lake Euphemia as the sun set, listening to the resident swans quarreling with the invading flock of Canada geese. We spoke about his father's illness and how Matt might not have made the same decisions for himself. We also spoke about what Matt calls "emotional armor," a protective shield that allows him to practice medicine yet remain relatively unscathed.

> Physicians develop an emotional armor, where you have to make difficult decisions but not feel their impact directly. When we are dealing with patients, we are trained to be objective, to avoid intensity of emotions and anguish. When things are going badly, it is not in our best interest to be overwhelmed by feelings. We have to remain sharp and have good reflexes and sound judgment.
>
> The very first patient a doctor ever works with in the first year of medical school is a cadaver. There's a reason behind that training. It makes it possible for us to look at the human body as simply a system of organs. Right from the start, we are trained that way, before we ever really see or interact with our first patient. We are desensitized so that we can withstand the painful things we will encounter with respect to our patients and their suffering.
>
> When I am in the office and I know that somebody is experiencing devastating problems because of what has happened with their reaction to treatments, I can look at those situations objectively. I can sympathize with how they feel, but I am not truly experiencing what they feel.
>
> The emotional armor we develop is a bit like anesthesia. It is an intentional numbing that allows us to undertake stressful, challenging tasks and complete them. Each physician has his or her own amount of self-preservation, but I think that even my most empathetic colleagues have learned to create barriers.
>
> As a doctor, I can walk through my clinic that might be filled with difficult, anguishing situations, but I am wearing my armor suit. I can navigate through and remain an effective physician. When it is your own family member, the armor doesn't work. It's gone. Suddenly you're overwhelmed with feelings and aware of the consequences of each decision.
>
> When something happens to a family member or a close friend, it is

as though a match has been dropped inside my suit of armor. For the first time, I am feeling the burning pain of what is happening in the world.

Most unsettling to Matt are situations where he feels the anguish of a patient or family member so intimately that he cannot protect himself.

One evening, I saw a woman in her mid-thirties who came into the hospital with a headache. She was diagnosed with a large lung cancer and dozens of metastatic deposits in her brain, and she had never been a smoker. It came as a complete shock to her. The oncologist and I both went into her room and started sharing with her what we were finding and what it meant for her, objectively laying things out in a kind but dispassionate way.

We'd had this talk with other patients a lot over the years, and as we were getting to the point of talking to her about her prognosis, which was just going to be months, the hospital door flew open and three excited little girls ran into the room carrying cards and signs, and they jumped onto her bed. They were carrying get-well signs for their mom, and she turned to them and just completely turned her attention away from us. She smiled and beamed at her kids, thanking them.

The oncologist and I excused ourselves and stepped out in the hallway. I have three daughters at home, and the woman in the bed was very similar to my wife. That was a situation in which I was actually feeling the impact of what I was doing. The emotional armor, which normally protects me from pain, was pierced.

While I had never heard the term "emotional armor" before, this captured an essential component of the struggle between engagement/empathy and overexposure that physicians experience. Matt couldn't avoid the emotionally wrenching experience of meeting the dying woman's children as they jumped excitedly on her bed. He saw his wife and his own family. The distance disappeared. All he could do was to excuse himself, an interloper, from the room and leave the woman to enjoy her closeness with her children.

But how, I wondered, could Matt continue to expose himself to such raw emotion? Didn't this exact a heavy toll? A lot of people's exposure to oncology is through tragedies in their own families, he said, and they assume that oncologists are going from one tragedy to the next.

The truth is that most of oncology is taking care of a patient who has had a curative surgical procedure, and I am stepping in to provide an adjuvant therapy to prevent a recurrence of a cancer. After I am finished with their treatment each day, they go off to work or resume their day. A lot of the things that we treat are not terribly challenging or emotionally heart-wrenching.

That being said, there's the other 20 percent of patients who are not going to do well. The treatments are simply designed to improve their quality of life, such as to reduce the pain in a spot where the cancer has invaded into a bone. Even though that is a tragic situation for that patient and their family, what they express to me is appreciation. In the clinic, they are immensely grateful to our staff, because what we are doing often is exactly what they need. Most days, it is not emotionally wrenching to be an oncologist.

This is also true in my world as a neurosurgeon. While I take care of patients who are dying, the majority are not. A typical neurosurgical patient is one who is suffering from excruciating pain because of a ruptured intervertebral disc in either the neck or the low back. Most recover without surgery and benefit from physical therapy and sometimes injections. Surgery, when necessary, is often extremely gratifying for surgeon and patient alike, as the end result is relief from searing pain and restoration of function. While risk is a feature of any surgical procedure, these interventions and episodes of care are rarely life-threatening and usually relatively uneventful.

Moments of great intensity do occur regularly. How we handle them helps to define our relationships with our patients and with ourselves. Do we connect emotionally, or do we defend ourselves, protected by our armor? I remember moments that offered the potential for connection with a patient or family—moments where I fell short. Those have stuck with me over many years. I regard them as failures. Most physicians remember their failures far longer than they do their successes.

One such failure occurred early in my career, while I was a chief resident. I helped my attending, Donald Ross, a compassionate and technically adept neurosurgeon, remove a brain tumor from deep within the brain of a man in his early thirties. The surgery took many hours.

It went well, but we knew the patient's prognosis was extremely poor: initial pathology suggested a glioblastoma, a malignant brain tumor with a terrible life expectancy. Donald invited me to speak with the family in the consultation room after the surgery, while he stood by. Entering the cramped room, I encountered, for the first time, his wife, parents, and three small children, who nervously awaited our report.

I was scared and couldn't bring myself to tell them the truth, that this tumor was incurable, that the patient would die relatively soon. Instead, I parsed my words. They were technically correct, but avoidant. I didn't know it at the time, but I had donned emotional armor to shield myself from the feelings that flooded me when I stepped into the consultation room. Overwhelmed, I found their situation unbearably sad and had no idea how to face them. I also had a young wife and a small child. The patient and I were almost the same age. What he and his family needed were honesty and compassion. Instead, I avoided connecting, leaving someone else to fill in the gaps. Of course, there is no telling whether the next doctor would be any less avoidant of the dismal reality they were now confronting, but to this day, I carry a sense of failure: I avoided my own pain but fell short as a physician.

For all the formal training I received in the technical aspects of neurosurgery, I had none in its human aspects. These include communication skills such as discussing prognosis with a patient, delivering bad news, counseling patients on which treatments to take. To the extent that I learned such things, it was through observation of the attending and senior resident surgeons. No one ever discussed the emotional impact of a case, or the sadness we felt with the death of a patient. I never spoke with Dr. Ross about how I felt regarding the patient's family; looking back I believe he would have been receptive if only I had found the courage.

While our entire training program painstakingly enumerated complications in weekly Morbidity and Mortality Conference, we never talked about the impact a particular case had on us or shared the way we felt knowing we had caused a complication that might have led to a patient's injury or even his death. It was up to us to find our own way through those experiences. These behaviors led to the accretion of thicker emotional armor: with no formal training in how to manage the emotional impact of our job on ourselves and others, this became a necessary, reactive survival tool.

Another problem with medical training is that physicians are generally quite poor communicators. Dr. Mary Buss, chief of Palliative Care at Harvard Deaconess, observes that surgeons receive excellent technical educations but are poorly trained in communicating with patients and families. They have virtually no education or practice in discussing the withdrawal of life-sustaining treatments, and these conversations often occur without supervision. "Physicians," she says, "are terrible in assessing their own communication skills."

As physicians, do we connect emotionally or do we defend ourselves? We cultivate detachment and emotional distance as a coping mechanism against the pain of grief, loss, and failure. Yet our attempts to protect ourselves ultimately intensify feelings of loss and deprive us of resolution. I have come to see that these unresolved feelings contribute directly to professional burnout.

Before Victoria's illness, I didn't even realize I was doing this. Since then, I have come to recognize the armor doesn't ultimately serve me and is in fact a liability. Once I understood how it interfered with the intensity of my perceived experiences, I saw it as a hindrance, blocking emotional connections I have come to cherish. Removing the armor requires deliberate effort. Admitting to mistakes and feelings is difficult and feels unnatural at first, but in the end, it is liberating.

Dr. Buss notes that physicians are afraid of, and avoid, feelings of sadness. We reason, mistakenly, that being open to pain and loss could damage us; we fear losing our composure and appearing vulnerable. Yet accepting vulnerability is what most closely connects us with our patients. This is what they remember in the end, after all the tests and treatments are done. Patients crave acceptance, appreciation, and acknowledgment; we all want this for ourselves.

It intrigues me that compassion fatigue does not come from exposure to too much sadness. If it did, then palliative care physicians would be the least happy and most burned out physicians of all, yet in reality, they are some of the most satisfied of any specialty. It is not exposure to sadness that is the problem, but the way we respond to it and how we are affected by it. By opening ourselves to experiencing heartache, we allow ourselves to become more vulnerable.

Brené Brown describes the importance of allowing ourselves to be vulnerable and holds up the surgeon as an example of someone who is exempted from this by the technical nature of their work. Yet, as I have come to appreciate, it turns out no one gets a pass. Surgeons and pilots, those whose work requires high levels of technical skill with direct responsibility for the lives of others, have to be able to flex, operating at different levels of vulnerability, but the ability to access their vulnerability is still crucial. Doing so connects them with the privilege and seriousness of their enterprise.

Surgeons who try to reduce surgery to a purely technical exercise flounder as physicians. The best surgeons maintain their humanity and their vulnerability. The opposite—a pose of distance and imperviousness—leads us to dehumanize and objectify patients and is a recipe for disaster. We can see the pitfalls of this behavior everywhere in medicine. Mechanical metaphors abound in surgery. "He's a machine" is an admiring way to describe a colleague who puts aside his own needs and feelings to work unflaggingly. "Productivity" refers to doing lots of surgery and generating revenue. But these descriptions dehumanize both physician and patients: A person who is a machine is one who is not feeling. Productivity is a reflection of the diminishment of the patient: no longer a human being in need of help, the patient has been reduced to a body part in need of repair and assigned a monetary value.

Dehumanizing patients can lead to indifference in physicians. It is a privilege to be trusted to take care of every patient we encounter, yet we can lose sight of this and begin to see our patients as a burden, or as units of work, rather than as individuals. When people cease to matter, we cease to care. This is the precipice of burnout and invites mistakes and poor behavior, such as cutting corners or pushing the envelope by exposing patients to excessive risks.

Often, physicians hold themselves to unachievable standards of perfection. No surgery is ever perfect, yet we expect perfection from ourselves and from our colleagues. Partly the result of training, these unrealistic standards also interfere with emotional connection or empathy. Complications are an inevitable part of the work we do, yet physicians often lack self-compassion. We tend to be unforgiving of ourselves (and of our colleagues). Self-compassion is a crucial component of emotional flexibility; unrelenting self-criticism does not promote learning or modification of maladaptive behaviors.

As the brother of a patient, I discovered how it felt to be on the receiving end of care lacking in compassion and became determined to connect more deeply with my patients and my own emotions. Yet I wondered, how could I balance connection and detachment as a neurosurgeon? Did engaging emotionally with my patients mean I could no longer detach enough to be an effective surgeon? Would it be better to become a technician and leave the emotions to others?

I found the solution to this conundrum through a conversation with Helen Riess, author of *The Empathy Effect*. Dr. Riess explains that through the process of self- and other-empathy, emotional armor can be replaced by "emotional agility." Intrigued, I went on to read Susan David's *Emotional Agility*, which characterizes this healthier stance.

A key to developing emotional agility is a willingness to embrace our vulnerability. Emotional agility enables us to move easily between powerful emotions, recognizing feelings without becoming bogged down by them, to move fluidly through the demands of life without becoming stuck or overwhelmed. Emotionally agile people are dynamic:

They derive power from facing, not avoiding, difficult emotions, recognizing that "life's beauty is inseparable from its fragility." Thus, physicians become better able to connect more deeply with our patients and ourselves, increasing our satisfaction and engagement while staving off burnout. Achieving emotional agility gave Dr. David "the power of facing into, rather than trying to avoid, difficult emotions."

In my own life, I have discovered that the tremendous power of emotional connection is an antidote for compassion fatigue, burnout, and despair. This has meant becoming more flexible and resilient. By being less defended, I have become more, rather than less, available. But make no mistake, this requires constant effort. Just as with the emotional armor of practicing physicians, we all use defenses against perceived threats—as David illustrates in her book, our natural inclination is away from agility. By "unhooking," "showing up," and "stepping out," we put aside these maladaptive defenses and create new, and ultimately self-reinforcing, patterns of behavior. The pleasure of seeing with greater clarity and the creation of meaningful connections are their own reward. I liken the feeling of this transition to going from seeing in black-and-white to suddenly seeing in color: the increased richness is intoxicating and becomes its own reward. I don't want to go back.

Dr. Riess has studied the neurobiology of empathy, as outlined in *The Empathy Effect*. "Some people must turn down the dial on their emotional empathy to become objective enough to do their jobs. Think of firefighters, or surgeons, who must focus on the technical tasks to complete a successful operation and not be distracted until the operation is complete." She has created a validated program to increase empathy through training for medical practitioners, based on increasing the perceptual awareness of others centered on the seven keys of "E.M.P.A.T.H.Y." In this acronym, E stands for "eye contact"; M for "muscles of facial expression"; P for "posture"; A for "affect"; T for "tone of voice"; H for "hearing the whole person"; and Y for "your response."

Not only do practitioners need to be trained to have increased empathy and awareness of self and others, they also need to learn how to move between different states of empathetic responses with patients, as the need arises. Dr. Riess observes that:

> . . . emotional empathy must also be kept in balance with self-regulation to help manage excessive loads of emotional arousal that can lead to blurred boundaries and personal distress. If you are exposed to too much pain and suffering every day, such as a day in the life of an oncologist or social worker or prison guard, excessive emotional empathy can lead to depression, anxiety, and burnout. The sharp edge of empathy would soon become dull, and you'd start to distance yourself from the human experience. In the medical profession, we call this "compassion fatigue."

Emotional agility allows the surgeon to operate with dispassionate objectivity one moment and move toward intimate connection the next, as the situation demands. Without emotional agility, these transitions can be difficult to make.

Dr. Alan Davidson, an ER attending, was a colleague of mine for over twenty years. He had recently retired. One Saturday while I was on call, he presented to the ER as a patient, with right-sided numbness. Initially designated "code stroke," a CT scan instead suggested a brain tumor. An MRI suggested a glioblastoma, so I was consulted. I fearfully faced my friend, upset for him and his wife. When I told them the likely diagnosis, he replied, "Well, then I'm going to die, aren't I?" We both knew his prognosis was poor.

Aware that he entrusted me with his life, I took him to surgery a few days later. I warned him he might be more numb or weak after the procedure. When he awoke, Alan and I were pleased that he was no worse than before his operation. The postoperative MRI scan showed we had removed almost the entire tumor.

I met with Alan, his wife, and his son when the pathology results came back. I sat on the edge of his bed and told him his diagnosis. Neither of us was surprised by the results. But he choked up as he expressed gratitude for his care. Holding back tears, I told him I felt honored he trusted me enough to take care of him. In the past, I would never have allowed myself to acknowledge my gratitude to Alan or the depths of his gratitude to me: I would have truncated the conversation and pushed these feelings away. We spoke for quite a while until I had to return to the operating room for another case.

As I left, Alan noted that my work seemed to fill me with energy and joy. I was surprised to realize I did not feel depleted, but rather that I felt privileged to witness both the beauty and fragility of life. At that moment, I knew I had discarded my irreparably damaged suit of emotional armor. In its place I had substituted something far more powerful: emotional agility.

Later, Alan was readmitted to the hospital with increasing numbness on his right side. I read him a draft of an essay I was writing about him. He sat in his bed, unable to control his phone or computer, yet emotionally attuned and intellectually forceful. He was pleased; he wanted me to tell his story. He felt strongly this message must be shared, agreeing that doctors often are burdened by perceived failures and private grief.

As we sat together, we reminisced about his life. We spoke of his worries for his wife, children, and grandchildren. He told me of professional mistakes that haunted him, yet he also spoke proudly of the thousands of patients he had cared for. Their individual stories and faces were no longer distinct but flowed through him. Just as Alan needed to recognize and admit his failings, he also needed to let them go. This is true for all of us: we must celebrate our victories, admit our failings, and forgive ourselves and each other. The connections we established did us both a world of good; he needed them, as did I.

I have described emotional armor, truncated communications, and barriers to emotional connection from the physician's point of view. But how does this feel to the patient? Through speaking with my sister and later from reading her journal, I learned what it felt like to be on the receiving end of these kinds of communication. Fear and a profound desire for connection were driving forces for Victoria. Most of her interactions with her physicians were positive, yet some communications increased her fear and her anxiety, causing her considerable stress. Two experiences stand out in her journal entries. The first was from a legalistic physician explaining the risks of different types of radiation to kill off her bone marrow in preparation for her bone marrow transplant. This was extremely frightening for Victoria, who didn't want to hear details, but instead wanted support, of which she felt little.

> Once I found my way to radiation, I found myself wondering how I could possibly have requested this particular method! The consult began with chatting with one somewhat junior doctor about the efficacy of targeted vs. whole-body radiation, and I couldn't follow a darn thing he said. I don't think it was me. It was a circuitous, utterly confusing discussion. After what felt like half an hour, I heard him say, "The TMI vs. TBI [I believe that is total marrow irradiation, versus total body irradiation] was likely no worse and possibly better re: secondary cancers." I felt like I was talking to a "lawyerdoc" or a "docyer."   —MARCH 21, 2015

Earlier, she described how terrified she was upon being transferred from St. John's, where she felt supported, to City of Hope, which felt harsh and clinical in comparison. Her intake interview, which occurred late in the evening after a long day of travel through snarled traffic on LA freeways, did not inspire comfort. That the admitting doctor referred to her previous treatment as a "failure" caused her to doubt the care she had received previously and made her feel that it was somehow her fault. She described her reactions to that discussion in her journal, which I cited in the chapter on her diagnosis.

But Victoria spoke and wrote about Dr. Fischer in glowing terms. She did not feel judged by him but reveled in his positivity. She adored him.

> When talking with Dr. Fischer, he once again, reminded me that he is CONFIDENT I'm going to do great—that I have so much going for me: intelligence, determination, an amazing support team, my family and friends. He also remarked how not everyone does anywhere near as well as I have done with the ARA-C. He said the transplant will not be a cakewalk but he is certain I'm going to do great.

This would horrify Dr. Fischer but several of us agreed that he is the real "Dr. McDreamy." He is an excellent doctor, who happens to be highly attractive. And he is a kind man. I was listening to an interview with Dr. Bernie Siegel talking about how many doctors go into medicine because they are interested in the science aspect, less the idea of working with patients. Dr. Fischer does both and he would never call my chemo a "fail!" In fact, he said he would have preferred the term "sub-optimal," which delivers a very different message, one of hope, not of failure . . . From the very beginning, he set a positive picture in place and I have followed his lead.

When he first told me I had leukemia, he said, "This is life-threatening but not a death sentence." That was very clear and an upbeat way to look at it. The message being: this will be hard, you have your work cut out for you, but you can do this. He has never wavered in his support. Even when I was at City of Hope, he was emailing me, seeing how I was doing and he'd always finish with, "You're going to do great." One time, I commented that perhaps the supplements I took with regularity have helped me do so well. He replied, "Or maybe it's just you." —FEBRUARY 21, 2015

When I spoke with Dr. Fischer, I told him I struggled with the implications of her diagnosis and how to relay this to Victoria, who made it clear to me that she did not wish to talk about dying or the concept of her own mortality. I wondered how this had affected the difficult conversations he had with Victoria and Pat and if he had also found it challenging.

After doing this for some time, and you probably know this yourself, you deal with each individual differently. I felt like Victoria's personality type was one I was familiar with. Such individuals thrive on the positive and avoid the negative. I felt like she wanted as little information as possible so that she could focus on the kind that would help her achieve very short-term goals.

"Hey, what can we do to get my bone marrow into remission? What can we do to mitigate side effects? What can we do to allow me to get home faster?" My understanding in speaking with her was always that she got it. It wasn't that she didn't want to know. She did know, but she didn't want to acknowledge it in her mind because it would take her to a dark place. I think she needed that positive energy to hold on to, and to get her through the day-to-day, week-to-week struggle of all of the treatment and the side effects, and the dealing with having young kids.

There were times where we would sit down and she would let that guard down and say, "Look, this is what we are going to have to do." I think she would take it in and kind of reset and start again where she would focus on short-term things, and not start thinking about transplants and donors. I think it was more, "All right, so I am going to have my bone marrow next week. Okay, I am going to stay positive and hope that my bone marrow is negative, and hope that I don't need a platelet transfusion tomorrow, and hope that I don't get nausea or vomiting . . ." We focused a lot less on the big picture with her, at least up front.

With Victoria, I viewed it as purely a defense mechanism. She needed to be strong for her children. I think everybody is different in how they approach it, and this was something that she created for her own mental well-being as a barrier to insulate herself, and maybe say to Pat, "You deal with some of these bigger things like insurance issues, and scheduling, and appointments, and visitors, and family." She told me, "I am going to focus on what I can do immediately, short-term."

She got it, she understood, and I think it wasn't denial. I think it was acceptance, but it was a very muted acceptance. She understood the gravity of the situation. She understood that it was a very serious, potentially life-threatening disease. Once she acknowledged that, she did not want to revisit it: "We are not going there again. We are going to take care of business. We are going to get to the place where I have the best opportunity to be cured and focus on all things positive." And that is what she did.

I asked Sean to take me through Victoria's transplant from his perspective.

When I first got that piece of information about her diagnosis, I was quite upset. I didn't verbalize that I was upset, and I didn't go into a lot of the immediate specifics about it, other than to say gingerly, "This may be something that we have to get you to a transplant center to discuss."

As time went on, I reinforced that a little bit more, and now instead of the word "may," the words "when you are scheduled" were what I used. I was communicating with Dr. O'Donnell at City of Hope. When I saw that prognostic feature come back, [I knew] that [Victoria's] only chance at this point would be a successful transplant, barring any scientific breakthrough.

While I recognized that the possibility of relapse and failure was there, among our discussions it was understood that this was certainly no guarantee for a cure. This would be the only shot of long-term survival. I tried not to get into the weeds with percentages. . . . because she did not ask me. If she had asked, I would have told her, but I felt—again, that theme of short-term goals—it was my job to try to get her prepared. To use a sports analogy, I was the starting pitcher, and I was trying to get her to the closer. My job was just to keep the game in check until we were able to get her to City of Hope, to the ultimate therapy that would give her the best chance. It was week to week, month to month, the kind of goals that we are talking about.

I wondered how he manages the stress and the grief that come with his job. Did he think that sustained exposure to loss leads to physician burnout, and did he and his medical community take any steps to prevent burnout, which is currently estimated to affect 55 percent of physicians?

It is a major struggle. I think of the good: we cure so many people. We do well by so many patients, and there is so much positive energy that comes out of that aspect of the practice. You deal with people [whom] you get to know intimately. You know their families and their family dynamics. I feel like I go to work and I open myself up, and then when I leave, I have a family and four kids, and I have to turn it off. I have been able to do that.

You find an outlet. Exercise has always been a big outlet for me, and music, and things that take my mind away from the morbid details, but it is a real challenge. That is why there is such a high burnout rate in the oncology profession.

It is well-known in the field that there are lots of issues with physician substance abuse and doctors ending their careers abruptly because they can't handle the stress. Actually, because of several cases of physician-reported substance abuse, there is a grief counseling program at the hospital. I don't think many doctors use it. I know that because the grief counselor is a patient of mine. There is clearly a need, but I think people are reluctant to do it.

I think there are people [who] benefit from this kind of grief counseling. I can only speak for myself and say that the initial part of my career was challenging. I would take a patient's death very personally from a professional standpoint, but also, I would have a hard time losing someone I cared about. I hate to say it, but over time, I think there has been a gradual numbing to this effect, where I now understand that I had nothing to do with the development of illness, that this was going to happen whether these people [had] ever met me or not.

I give them the best opportunity to get on the right path toward cure or palliation, but if my patient succumbs to their illness, I have learned to accept that while I am sad, I also understand that this is the cycle. Until there are major breakthroughs in the field, which hopefully will be coming soon, it is going to be this way.

I spoke with Sean about Matt Manning's concept of emotional armor and wanted to know what steps he takes to avoid becoming overwhelmed by his job.

> There is just not enough time in the day. You will see one more patient and you don't get off until 10 p.m. There are doctors [who] do that every day, at the expense of themselves. With my own responsibilities to my family, I can't do that. I feel an obligation to do both, so I try very hard to do everything I can for patients while I am here, and there are certain people, Victoria being one of them, for whom I will respond to an email or provide my cell phone [number], which I don't do frequently. Just knowing that I am available is a major boost for patients.

In his own way, Sean has managed to come to terms with the emotional burdens of working as an oncologist and to balance his life as an engaged and vital human being. This is an example of emotional agility in action. I think he would probably say that it hasn't been easy getting to this place, but he has successfully avoided the pitfalls of burnout and walling himself off emotionally. He can only do so much; he has accepted and come to terms with his limitations.

Gus Magrinat has adopted a similar balance. When I spoke with him about denial and how he chooses what information to share with his patient, his stance also reflects his own emotional agility. He begins by asking the patient what questions he or she might have.

> If they say, "I want to know everything," I say, "What other questions do you have?" If they do not ask, "How long am I going to live?" or "Is this curable?" then I know that they do not want to talk about it. My job is still to convey important information, and so what I say in stage IV cases is "You know, I do not like to tell you this, but it is important to me that you understand we do not know how to cure this disease at this point. We may know how to cure it in two years or five years, but today we cannot. So, the goal of treatment cannot be cure." I leave it there.
>
> Now, if the patient does ask, then I can give them a lot more

information, and I always give the information as numerically as possible. "You have a fifty-fifty chance of being alive in six months. That is a very important thing for me to be able to say, because it qualifies you for hospice if you want to participate in hospice. Legally, that is important, but that does not mean you are going to live six months, and it does not mean that you are going to be dead in six months. It's just a statistical thing." So, I have those discussions.

I don't feel it's my job to hit them over the head with facts. I let them know the situation, and if they deny it, then that's their choice. It is a problem for the families. They lie to the families. "My doctor said that I'm fine." "I take my treatments, and everything is going well." Then the family is in shock to hear she's got five days. She knows it, but she doesn't tell them.

I would translate it this way: "I know I'm going to die, but I don't want to deal with it. I'm not denying, because denial means I'm not sick." Denial is more like "I don't need treatment. Why would I get treatment? I'm not sick.'" No. They're not denying in the sense that they refuse treatment or don't understand. They understand and do get treated, but they really don't want to face it. They don't want to discuss that. There are many ways of doing that. One of these [ways] is to say, "I'm going to be fine. Treatment's great, and it's working, and . . . I'm not worried." Whatever their statement is, what it really means is "I don't want to look at it."

When physicians discard their self-protective stance, the result is richer relationships, greater connections with patients, and less burnout and compassion fatigue. Emotional agility is a far healthier strategy, and physicians need to embrace it through training, support, and community. Paradoxically, the answer to burnout and compassion fatigue is more, rather than less, compassion. In a way, Victoria's denial of her own mortality was a form of self-protection similar to the emotional armor physicians adopt, although clearly from Scan Fischer's perspective, it was far more nuanced than I realized. But her unwillingness to accept conflicting narratives and to balance between them did reflect a lack of emotional agility. Emotional agility would have allowed her to move between immediate treatment objectives and a wider picture of her disease. Just as physicians fail when they lack agility, she denied herself and her family the opportunity to say goodbye in the face of her leukemia recurrence and almost certain death.

Patients make better decisions with more, rather than less information. Doctors and nurses navigate healthcare with greater ease than do patients without medical backgrounds. Partly, this reflects greater comfort with the complex and often nonintuitive systems of hospitals and medical care, but it also comes from familiarity with the science and medical basis for making the best possible decisions. The better informed patients are, the better the decisions they will make for themselves and their family members. It is helpful for patients to understand their situations and options to the best of their abilities rather than to blindly trust their doctors and medical teams. This is why education and preparation are so important. People need to make advance directives and difficult decisions before they are confronted with catastrophic illness, not during the tumult that ensues.

As Victoria's journal and reactions to her care illustrate, the onset of a major health crisis is not always the best moment to become an educated patient, as she was in the grip of fear. Both Gus Magrinat and Sean Fischer have struggled with how much to tell their patients and how to deliver bad news. They have come to remarkably similar approaches: they follow the patient's lead by giving as much information as he or she wants. They have learned that "hitting them over the head" doesn't work. Sean worked within Victoria's capacity to handle medical information and provided the optimism and support he rightly felt she craved. Emotional agility is an essential element for patients and practitioners alike in achieving a balance between the intense emotions they are suddenly experiencing and the ability to draw on the many resources that are available to them for the asking.

enhancing palliative care: asking for a most benevolent outcome

To cure sometimes, to relieve often, to comfort always.
—EDWARD LIVINGSTON TRUDEAU

Early involvement of palliative care is essential in facilitating honest conversations and considering transitioning to less intensive treatments. In patients with advanced cancers, earlier consultation with palliative care, rather than waiting until the disease has even further progressed, leads to improved symptom and pain management, clarification of goals of care, and medically appropriate decision-making. This has been shown to lower costs, increase satisfaction in patients and their families, and shift care away from hospitals to home settings. Efforts to invite earlier consultation have proven effective, such as changing the name to "supportive care," thereby avoiding the stigma often associated with the name "palliative care"; pushing palliative care upstream into the clinic; or the institution of Baylor's doula program, in which trained volunteers provide support to dying patients.

Physicians are frequently reluctant to involve palliative care services for their patients, typically referring only late in an illness. Seventy percent of doctors state they have no training in palliative care, and many do not understand the distinction between palliative care and hospice care. They are reluctant to involve palliative care because they believe this is only appropriate within six months of anticipated death of the patient; whereas, in fact, palliative care can be invoked at the time of diagnosis. Palliative care is an interdisciplinary effort to improve the quality of life of patients of any age who have been diagnosed with a serious illness, as well as the lives of their families. Amy Kelley, MD, writing in the *New England Journal of Medicine* in 2015, defines the core components of palliative care as "the assessment and treatment of physical and psychological symptoms, identification of and support for spiritual distress, expert communication to establish goals of care and assist with complex medical decision making, and coordination of care."

Doctors frequently do a poor job of assessing a patient's overall circumstances, either because they do not have the time or because they do not consider this valuable information. Demographic factors like age, sex, and marital status are straightforward, but often the parts of a patient's narrative that may profoundly inform decision-making and treatment outcomes remain unexplored.

The social aspects of patients' lives are every bit as important as the medical ones. For many years, I have cared for a now-middle-aged man, Jake, who carries the diagnosis of Asperger's syndrome. Jake is socially withdrawn and has spent much of his life in an institution. He developed seizures, which led to the diagnosis of an intermediate-grade brain tumor (an oligodendroglioma), which we removed and for which he subsequently received radiation therapy. He did well with these treatments and went to live with his elderly mother. Every few months I would see him in our brain tumor clinic along with Matt Manning. Together, we addressed the medical issues of his care and concerns about

Jake's seizures, which occur infrequently and are well controlled with antiepileptic medications.

Early on, we embedded a palliative care nurse practitioner in our multidisciplinary brain tumor clinic. We have found that this service not only improves the quality of care but also, surprisingly, reduces costs as we shift toward less intensive care more in keeping with patient desires. After our last visit, Mary Larach, the nurse practitioner, met with Jake and his mother. After Mary reported her findings, both Dr. Manning and I realized how little we understood Jake's situation. Neither the tumor nor his seizures were their primary concern. His mother was terrified that she was becoming too old to care for Jake. His tenuous future kept her up at night, and she panicked about having to return her son to an institution he hated. Dr. Manning and I were focused on Jake's tumor, but this was the least of Emily's worries. In clinic, we tend to speak more than we listen. Mary, less concerned with a medical agenda, is freer to listen. Both aspects of care are important. The key is teamwork and the synthesis that comes with open communication.

Similarly, we recently cared for Leo, a young man with metastatic lung cancer to his brain, which we had treated with focused radiation (stereotactic radiosurgery). Leo seemed to be doing well after this treatment, regaining some of his energy and strength. He worked high up on storage tanks, cleaning them with toxic solvents. Dr. Manning and I both advised him to quit this job for the time being. Leo's balance was impaired, and we were afraid that he would fall from one of these tanks and be seriously injured. What neither of us grasped was the impact of Leo's home situation on his treatment decisions. He understood he had lung cancer and was not afraid to die. It turns out that he has five children, all from different mothers, and owes child support for each of them. He was convinced that he would go to jail if he stopped paying child support. The money he would receive from disability if he stopped working would not begin to cover his financial obligations, let alone his personal expenses. The brain tumor was a sideshow to his more pressing concerns.

Palliative care services have grown 150 percent in the last few years but are still unevenly available in the United States. There are regional disparities (more common in the Northeast than in the South), disparities related to the size of hospitals (more common in larger hospitals with more than 300 beds than in smaller hospitals), and also disparities based on socioeconomic and racial status of patients. Not only is there a lack of training and awareness of the value of palliative care services for patients among all doctors, but also there is a shortage of palliative care physicians across the United States. Palliative care services are often available in hospitals, but there is an unmet need among the 1.8 million patients in long-term-care facilities and among those patients who are treated in outpatient settings in the community.

Awareness of the importance of palliative care has improved in the management of patients with fatal or relentlessly debilitating diseases, such as cancer and dementia. Increased availability of these services has led to decreased in-hospital deaths and better communication with patients and their families, but palliative care is not as widely available in many chronic diseases, such as kidney failure, pulmonary diseases, and heart failure. The rates of in-hospital death and the involvement of palliative care services lags behind in these diagnoses.

How Victoria faced her diagnosis of AML, choosing life over death and opting for aggressive treatment despite long odds, is, surprisingly, a typical reaction to this catastrophic diagnosis. A Duke University study discusses the impact of a diagnosis of AML on thirty-two newly diagnosed patients, who were interviewed. "Four main themes emerged: (a) shock and suddenness, (b) difficulty processing information, (c) poor communication, and (d) uncertainty. Patients frequently described their diagnosis as shocking. They also felt that the amount of information was overwhelming and too difficult to process, which negatively impacted their understanding. Patients frequently described a lack of emotional support from clinicians and described uncertainty about their prognosis, the number and nature of available treatments, and what to expect from treatment."

While AML is potentially curable in favorable groups or in younger patients, "high risk groups have a five year survival of under 10 percent, akin to that of metastatic pancreatic cancer. Despite this, patients with AML are often treated more aggressively than patients with advanced solid tumors, presumably due to the chance of cure. They are, therefore, less likely to use specialist palliative care or hospice services and are more likely to die in the hospital." The article goes on to describe how patients will often opt for more intensive therapies given in a hospital with higher risk of complication and death for the outside chance of a cure, rather than less intensive therapies as an outpatient. Patients diagnosed with AML face unique stresses, due both to the frequent need to be transferred to academic centers far from their homes and the rapidity of the illness, the latter necessitating "a compressed timeline in which to make decisions." They are often overwhelmed by the suddenness of the diagnosis and frequently "dichotomize treatment options into either 'do or die,' when there [are] actually several available treatment options of varying intensity and risk."

Many patients "described a mismatch between their informational needs and the type of information physicians provided," which often resulted in their feeling dissatisfied. The authors conclude that "in an era where patients are supposed to be participating in 'shared decision making,' we found that many patients with AML do not even have a functional understanding of their disease or of the risks and benefits of available therapies," making shared decision-making "a particularly difficult challenge in the AML setting." According to the Duke study:

> Patients often described "abduction by the illness" and a subsequent surrendering of control to the medical system. . . . Older patients with AML often did not know their prognosis and many grossly overestimated their likelihood of survival at 6 months. . . . Many patients reported an expected cure rate of over 90%, wherein their oncologists estimated it at below 10%. . . . Many patients described blunt communication that lacked emotional support, resulting in feelings of disappointment, fear, or even abandonment. Oncologists often miss opportunities to empathize with

their patients, and our data suggest that this finding is true in the AML setting as well.

In this context, Victoria's reaction to her diagnosis and illness seem entirely consistent with this reported framework of how patients react to a new diagnosis of AML. In *When Blood Breaks Down*, Mikkael Sekeres supports this finding, citing "a separate study in 260 patients undergoing a bone marrow transplant found that those with higher-risk cancers—meaning that their expected survival following the transplant was lower—tended to be much more optimistic about their chances than their doctors." (p. 87) Prolonged hospitalizations and in-hospital deaths in patients with AML were the norm, rather than the exception. In one study of 330 people diagnosed with AML from 2005 to 2011, "those who died spent over 28 percent of their lives from the moment of diagnosis in the hospital and almost 14 percent in the clinic. Within 30 days of death, 85 percent were hospitalized, 45 percent had received some type of chemotherapy, and 61 percent died in the hospital." (p. 257)

The difference between the ways in which many doctors choose to end their own lives and how they prescribe treatment to others is telling. This speaks to difficulties with trust and the management of expectations of patients, as well as to better understanding of risks and benefits of treatment and comfort with medical decision-making among physicians. These inconsistencies are emblematic of the problems we have with discussing and understanding death in our society.

Several articles have highlighted these differences. Ken Murray's "How Doctors Die," looks at the choices some physicians made when they became patients and faced terminal illnesses. They opted for less care, rather than more, and usually chose to stay home, rather than go to the hospital. They accepted the consequences of their diagnosis and preferred to maximize quality-of-life considerations over quantity of life. Another article, "Association of Occupation as a Physician with Likelihood of Dying in a Hospital," by Saul Blecker et al., published in *JAMA* in 2016, analyzed the death certificates of physicians and similarly educated professionals and concluded, "Physicians were slightly less likely to die in a hospital than the general population, but equally as likely to die in a hospital as others in health care or with similar educational attainment. In addition, physicians were the least likely group to die at any facility." The authors state that this area is poorly studied and that an analysis of death certificates and place of death does not provide understanding of nuance or the choices patients make in their end-of-life care.

Ironically, by declining care, many terminally ill patients extended their remaining time longer than their treating physicians had anticipated they would live. This doesn't surprise me, because we tend to overestimate the benefits of the interventions we provide toward the end stages of a disease process. We downplay the risks and suffering so that avoidance of some care options, particularly when the likelihood of benefit is low, may end up helping the patient rather than causing harm, at least in the short-term. Certainly, the quality of a patient's remaining time is better with fewer drugs and fewer invasive treatments, and patients are often energized by doing things that give them pleasure and meaning. They surround themselves with family and friends, minimizing time in the hospital.

Dr. Sekeres provides data to support the observations that patients and doctors "exaggerate the benefits of interventions and minimize the harms. In one systematic review of 35 studies that enrolled over 27,000 patients, most participants overestimated benefit for 65 percent of outcomes, and underestimated harm for 67 percent . . . Doctors don't fare much better. In another systematic review of 48 studies that included more than 13,000 clinicians . . . more than half of the participants overestimated benefits, and underestimated harm, for almost one-third of outcomes." (p. 82)

Patients and their families often ask me, "What would you do if this were you or someone you love?" I am well aware that thinking about a situation in the abstract is different from living with a poor prognosis as a daily reality. The implication of a cancer diagnosis in my patients always gives me pause, yet when my sister was diagnosed with leukemia, my reaction was intense and raw. The distance I normally rely upon in order to make decisions and put plans into action had vanished, replaced by fear and emotional pain.

Should I become gravely ill, provided there were good treatment options, I would almost certainly pursue them. I would be willing to undergo surgery and accept physical pain if there were a high likelihood of success. Had I been in Victoria's position, I would also have willingly undergone a bone marrow transplant.

Because I am a physician, my relationship to my caregivers would be inherently different than my sister's. I lack her degree of faith and trust. Decisions would be made based on the knowledge and facts at our disposal, and I would want to be part of the process. I don't believe I would agree to treatment for lack of anything better; for example, I would likely have drawn a line after early recurrence of the leukemia posttransplant, since the likelihood of cure at that point was essentially nil.

Our culture has systematically removed death from everyday life. We avoid talking about it. As a result of this avoidance, 80 percent of Americans do not put their affairs in order before they die. The vast majority of Americans say they wish to die at home, but 75 percent die in a hospital or in a nursing home. This has begun to change: in 2017, 29.8 percent of deaths by natural causes occurred in hospitals and 30.7 percent occurred at home (Kolata, 2019). People who live alone, isolated from family and friends, have higher rates of admission and in-hospital death, even when those patients express the same desire to die at home as do patients with greater social support. Our relationships with others are a crucial part of the end of life. We need to strengthen these connections.

In their last month alone, half of Medicare patients go to an emergency department, one-third are admitted to an ICU, and one-fifth will have surgery—even though 80 percent of patients say they hope to avoid hospitalization and intensive care at the end of life. This is largely because patients are ill-prepared to confront their mortality and medical professionals are not willing to tackle the business of dying. Medicare spending for patients in the last year of life is six times what it is for other patients and accounts for a quarter of the total Medicare budget. This proportion has remained essentially unchanged for the past three decades, despite increasing awareness of the need for earlier discussion of issues surrounding end-of-life care.

Often, the first time people talk about death is in the doctor's office, when they may discover they are critically ill. If we engage in conversations about death long before we must face it, perhaps this will alleviate some of the fear, encourage us to live more fully, and allow us to prepare for our inevitable mortality. People want to go down swinging. I respect that desire, but not at the cost of denying reality. If Victoria had been able to acknowledge her predicament after her transplant failure, perhaps she might have done things differently those last few weeks of her life. So often, an unwillingness to confront our mortality is a kind of magical thinking from which no good comes. We miss opportunities to say and do what we really want, and instead, we may spend our remaining days stranded in a disorienting fog of treatments and their side effects.

It is important to know a patient's goals, fears, and expectations. Atul Gawande addresses this constellation in *Being Mortal*. A patient may be married, but the marriage may be an unhappy one. They may be fearful of the financial consequences of prolonged illness or treatment. They may be scared of death or accepting of dying. Some patients say they are ready to die, and older patients in particular, those who have already lost loved ones and friends, may themselves have lost interest in living and welcome death, rather than wishing desperately to prolong their lives.

The opposite is true of someone like my sister, who was in the prime of her life and desperately wanted to live. The degree of acceptance of a terminal diagnosis is often colored by the quality of life that the patient has lived to date and the level of personal satisfaction they feel. It matters greatly whether the patient is in a critical, time-sensitive episode of illness, such as a brain hemorrhage, in which decisions need to be made immediately or in a slower-moving scenario, such as prostate cancer.

Of great importance is whether the patient is conscious and competent. I spend a lot of time with families who must suddenly care for loved ones after a severe injury resulting in impaired levels of consciousness. In these situations, families need to speak on behalf of the patient. They often struggle to reach consensus regarding care, particularly when it comes to withdrawal of treatment when the likelihood of meaningful survival is negligible. Rifts can build between family members, and long-seething resentments surface in strange and often unexpected ways. Estranged family members may be the most uncomfortable with discontinuing care; the loudest protests can come from those who do not actually show up at the hospital.

This is one reason that living wills are crucial, yet only approximately one in three adults in the United States has one. Honest discussions about your end-of-life wishes, sharing these wishes with loved ones now in case you become unable to express them later, make these excruciating circumstances easier to navigate. Of course, it is not possible to project every eventuality in a written document, but by talking about it beforehand, family members have a far better idea what their loved one would want and can act on those wishes. I spend considerable time explaining to families that the emphasis should not be on what they would desire for themselves but on the understanding that they are acting *as the voice of the impaired patient*. Their duty is to honor *the patient's* wishes as best they can.

One of the ironies that frequently plays out in the ICU is that patients and family members who have lived unhappy or unfulfilling lives will cling to life and demand that "everything be done," not realizing that by making these demands they are ensuring that the patient experiences a bitter end, remaining on a ventilator for a prolonged period of time or moving to a nursing home for the remainder of his or her days.

Sometimes, families of patients who have felt disenfranchised in their lives will demand heroic, aggressive intervention in the ICU and remain suspicious of any efforts made by the medical team to back off on treatments, no matter how futile those treatments may be. By contrast, those who have led fulfilling lives and have announced their wishes for the end of life in advance of a critical illness seem to anguish less over the medical decisions. More often, they choose graceful exits rather than prolonged and painful ones. In both instances, open communication with families is imperative. There is clearly a racial disparity between patient and family willingness to involve palliative care or hospice services and transition from more aggressive to less aggressive care. This includes frequency of in-hospital death, with African American patients more likely to die in the hospital than white patients. African American patients are more likely to mistrust the medical system and to avoid enrolling in hospice care than white patients. They are less likely than white patients to know about these care options, such as home hospice. Efforts are being made to ameliorate these disparities.

Ideally, both the patient and the physician should be united in a desire for authenticity and understanding. Familiarity with the real possibility of dying allows for trust and open communication, so that both parties can strive for honest connection. This is why it is important that we physicians understand a patient's idea of appropriate and compassionate care and why it is similarly essential that the physician be honest about the disease process, its likely outcomes, and the implications of treatment

As physicians, we need to communicate technical information to patients—biology, physiology, and treatment issues—including side effects and complications, whether they be related to surgical procedures, chemotherapies, drugs, or radiation therapy. We have to review tests, interpret data, counsel patients, and chart these interactions in excruciating detail. Adding on emotional support, such as grief counseling and details of palliative care, seems altogether too much for one individual to manage. We need to work seamlessly as a team, and health systems should be organized with an eye to this approach, with the goal of decreasing the burden on physicians and simultaneously improving patient care. Bringing palliative care services into play earlier in patients' illnesses, rather than waiting until the end of life, will not only improve the patient's experience but also off-load physicians. This needs to be strongly encouraged both in hospitals and medical practices. Not only will patients receive better care, but physicians will also feel less burdened, more supported by their health systems, and as Stacy Wentworth and Sean Fischer suggest, freed to address the many necessary aspects of patient care they are currently expected to manage.

Palliative care nurses have been an enormous benefit to brain tumor patients in our multidisciplinary cancer treatment program. Their involvement should be the rule, rather than the exception. In the Neuro-ICU at my hospital, involvement of palliative care is inconsistent and depends on who is attending a given patient, as well as frequently complex family situations. These observations are supported by Susan Shapiro's *Speaking for the Dying: Life-and-Death Decisions in Intensive Care*, in which she systematically observes on a daily basis how decisions are made in two ICUs in a diverse urban hospital. These decisions, and the quality of communication with patients and families, are highly variable and frequently unpredictable. Physicians who welcome the involvement of palliative care are often more sensitive to the issues that are affecting patients and their families, while others are less receptive to these concerns and may be unwilling to involve palliative care services in the first place. We have tried to eliminate this variability in our hospital by embedding palliative care services in the ICU, just as we have done so in the brain tumor clinic. While this effort has only recently been initiated, we believe this will make for greater patient and family satisfaction and is also likely to curtail unnecessary procedures and suffering. These interventions have been shown in other institutions to save money and to increase satisfaction.

Psychologists are also extremely useful members of the treatment team. Knowing that the emotional concerns of patients are being handled well allows me to concentrate on their medical care. This is an enormous benefit to the patient as well as to the staff. But many medical systems do not provide these services, as they do not see a direct financial benefit but only a cost, measured in full-time equivalents (FTEs), to these added staff. The cost-effectiveness of these services is changing as organizations transition from fee-for-service models to those based on population health, or to value-based care, in which health systems are responsible for the overall costs of care (earlier palliative care drives these down), as opposed to billing for interventions that are not necessarily efficacious but almost always expensive and profitable.

Physicians receive little support in the form of counseling, grief management, or ongoing professional training. Stacy Wentworth suggests that we return for training after completing residency and formal medical education. This could be accomplished through workshops and continuing education programs for physicians designed to reinforce skills and supplement our earlier formal medical training. These programs already exist, but they need to be made more widely available. Included should be training in interviewing techniques, becoming comfortable speaking with patients and their families about end-of-life care, and sharing the insights of palliative medicine with other specialties. In my practice, a significant portion of my time is spent conducting interviews, yet I have had no formal training in this and receive no feedback on my skills in this area. Most doctors learn as they go, with no training after medical school and residency have been completed, and because of this we are likely to repeat mistakes or miss opportunities to improve.

It is only after we have been in practice for several years that we begin to formulate new questions about, and insights into, patient care. There are few avenues for coaching or professional development available to physicians in practice. Perhaps some physicians do not see the need for ongoing training or grief counseling, but I think these services are beneficial, especially when we think of a doctor's exposure to tragedy and loss as cumulative. Partly, this is a cultural issue because just as patients and people in general don't discuss death or dying, physicians don't readily choose to discuss their failures and sadness. Medical systems don't invite this type of disclosure, and often doctors do so at their own risk. Administrators and peers may perceive such behavior as a sign of weakness or maybe "frailty," rather than a healthy way to grow as a practitioner and as a human being. Substance abuse, withdrawal, and failed marriages are well-known symptoms of burnout; these need to be prevented where possible and treated readily and without recrimination when they do occur.

compassion as a core value: improving the patient experience

Historically, physicians-in-training have been taught: "Don't get too close to patients." The thinking was that keeping a safe distance from patients—at least emotionally—would protect the caregiver by preventing emotional overextension and thus reduce the risk of getting burned out . . . the preponderance of data among health care providers actually shows the opposite to be true . . . the vast majority of published studies testing the association between compassion and burnout in health care providers found an *inverse* correlation. . . .That is, high compassion was associated with low burnout, and low compassion was associated with high burnout . . . these data do not support the historical thinking that too much compassion will burn you out. —STEPHEN TRZECIAK, MD AND ANTHONY MAZZARELLI, MD, *COMPASSIONOMICS*

We who work [in health care] are also unwitting agents for a system that too often doesn't serve . . . Because health care was designed with diseases, not people, at its center. —BJ MILLER, MD

A good physician treats the disease; the great physician treats the patient who has the disease. —WILLIAM OSLER, MD

Compassion is of vital importance in all areas of medicine, particularly surgery. Compassion means "to suffer with." It reflects the emotional response to another person's pain and involves an authentic desire to help. Not just the recipients, but also the givers of compassion can be affected in powerful ways. This is something we are rarely taught, often acculturating these values during our training. Empathy, our perception of others' emotions and perspectives, is essential for us to develop compassion. It has been shown that training can increase empathy in medical practitioners.

The opposite of compassionate care is transactional medical care. Maintaining the human connection between the patient and doctor, the bond of trust that carries through surgery and under general anesthesia, can be subverted by a relationship with the patient that discounts or eliminates the compassionate connection in favor of a transactional one. We see this when patients feel they have been objectified or that their doctors hold them in callous disregard. We see this when surgeons rush, cut corners, or recommend procedures based on the financial reward they provide. This is one of the problems inherent in the current cost and reimbursement structures of medical practice: we are encouraged to do more and are paid better the more procedures we perform.

In their book *Compassionomics,* Stephen Trzeciak and Anthony Mazzarelli show, with data, that a lack of compassion is often a learned behavior. While trainees may begin with empathy and compassion as core values, they often lose these during their training. Much of this occurs through the "hidden curriculum": "that which the school teaches without intending or being aware that it is being taught" (p. 18). For better or worse, trainees model their behavior on their mentors' examples, absorbing and imitating their approaches. As I discussed in Chapter Two, I trained under Buz Hoff at the University of Michigan. He fostered positive models of humanity and caring for both practitioners and patients. Other training programs may not be as supportive or may promote negative motivational models, which can include intimidation and fear.

We intuitively know that it is important for us to respect and feel compassion for our patients. But does this really matter? Are there data supporting the hypothesis that compassionate patient treatment produces better outcomes? Is the OR a place where compassion should be checked at the door? Or does compassion belong with our patients through their entire surgeries, exemplified by the surgeon and inculcated in the staff? There are actually very strong data supporting the importance of compassion in the operating room; better outcomes and greater patient safety are both strongly correlated with greater compassion.

Two of the main components of burnout are emotional exhaustion and depersonalization. Trzeciak and Mazzarelli provide evidence that "depersonalization and emotional exhaustion among surgeons were significantly associated with a higher incidence of major surgical errors." They go on to explain that depersonalization

> . . . involves objectifying patients as well as being uncaring and callous towards them . . . surgeons scoring high in emotional exhaustion (which leads to compassion fatigue) are prone to a lapse in clinical judgment that can result in major error. . . . Numerous other clinical studies have similarly supported that health care providers' inability to build meaningful relationships with patients can lead to low quality of care and is a risk to patient safety. For example, a Swiss study of 1,425 nurses and physicians working in ICUs found that emotional exhaustion—a precursor to compassion fatigue—among ICU staff was associated with higher ICU mortality. So, it's not just a higher error rate . . . it's a higher *death* rate. . . . lack of compassion among health care providers can be a serious patient safety risk. (p. 171)

Not only does greater compassion lead to better surgical outcomes and enhanced patient safety, it also decreases burnout in practitioners. Almost counterintuitively, our efforts to distance ourselves from the emotional impact of our work do us far more harm than if we accept both the grief and sadness that regularly accompany them.

The third main component of burnout is a sense of the lack of personal accomplishment or feeling that what you do doesn't make a difference. Greater compassion for and connection with our patients mitigates all three. The more we connect with our patients and express compassion, the better our patients fare and the more engaged we remain as practitioners. At the same time, operating with self-compassion allows us to forgive ourselves for the errors we may make. We are often our own harshest critics; when things do go wrong, our self-criticism can be withering and we lack the same kindness for ourselves that we try to show toward others.

Jodi Halpern explores the importance of empathic connections between doctors and their patients, including the philosophical and psychiatric basis for empathy, in *From Detached Concern to Empathy: Humanizing Medical Practice*. "The idea that accompanying patients in their suffering can be therapeutic leads to an alternative to the ideal of detached concern for patient-physician interactions." She describes the need to heal not just physical bodies but also patients' emotional states. "Emotional receptivity is needed if physicians are to acknowledge the pain and suffering that patients do not, and sometimes cannot put into words." (p. 145)

Dr. Halpern believes that empathy can be cultivated by helping "students develop and retain their engaged curiosity about other people's distinct experiences." She admits that this is difficult given the time pressures on physicians, the need to make rapid diagnoses, and the "pressure on physicians to know rather than to express uncertainty." As I suggested earlier, one way to counter the time pressures and expectations on physicians is to adopt a team approach to patient care and to encourage other members of the treatment team to foster empathic connections: "in practice, nurses, social workers, and other caregivers are frequently sources of empathy. Integrating empathy into medicine means including it in the entire team's approach." (p. 135)

Early in my practice, I tried to keep to medical subjects and facts when I spoke with my patients. Expressions of concern and compassion were permissible, but I consciously maintained a distance between us. Now, without the protection afforded by emotional armor, I am more aware of, and receptive to, the suffering of my patients. Perhaps it is because of sadness I feel about their frailty or loss, but I am also touched by their kindness and heroism. I have always been genuinely interested in their stories. William E. Williams, in the midst of his own struggle with brain cancer, brought me to tears when he asked about Victoria just after she died. When another patient, Stuart, heard about my sister's death, he stood up and spontaneously hugged me. Their compassion in the face of their own circumstances has taught me much about empathy and grace.

Christine came to my office with her elderly mother, Sarah, in tow. I had done surgery to remove pressure on Sarah's thoracic spinal cord in the hopes of restoring her ability to walk. I had operated on Christine's son, Maurice, many years earlier, removing a brain tumor, and she had thought so highly of me that she had brought her mother from Florida for her operation. The surgery had gone well from a technical standpoint, but Sarah did not regain the ability to walk and remained in a nursing home. As I spoke to Christine and Sarah, there was no recrimination, only sadness over what had been lost. Maurice had recently had a stroke and could no longer speak or walk. Christine's husband had died of cancer the year before. And now, her mother was wheelchair-bound and could no longer care for herself.

These losses have narrowed both women's existences and deprived Christine's mother of the connections and meaning that have been the basis for her daily life. She is no longer able to live independently at home and has lost the ability to perform simple activities we usually take for granted, such as dressing, using a toilet, or feeding herself. As I sat there and listened, I realized there was little I could do medically. I ordered an MRI to make sure there was no continued pressure on Sarah's spinal cord, but I told them it was unlikely I would be able to surgically fix the problem. Although Sarah might make some small improvements with continued rehabilitation and physical therapy, her weakness was most likely permanent. I asked about the nursing home and about Maurice's efforts toward speaking. I sat with them and listened to their stories, aware that their troubles were not fixable.

As a newly trained doctor, I would have been concerned about the medical facts, fearful Christine would somehow hold me responsible for Sarah's lack of improvement. I would have shown concern and sympathy, but then moved on to the next patient. As the three of us convened in my examination room, I didn't have an answer for their suffering. Yet our bond was powerful, and in a small way, perhaps it gave them comfort. For them to know that I cared, that I was sorry for their losses, that I would try to help them both as much as I could—that was the best I could offer.

I spoke with a good family friend, Sue Upton, whose experience illustrates the importance of strong communication between physicians and families. A clear grasp of the medical facts and being able to ask the right questions helped her family make optimal medical decisions. Several years ago, her father, Larry, died at Maine Medical Center as the result of herpes encephalitis, an illness that developed rapidly and robbed him of his intellectual powers, rendering him completely dependent on others. With his family's blessing, he died peacefully after the medical team transitioned from aggressive care to comfort care. Orchestrating his death in a way that felt dignified and complied with Larry's wishes required multiple conversations between the medical staff and his family.

When he was brought to the emergency department by ambulance, Sue's father was not conscious, and given the suddenness of his brain infection, he had not prepared any specific instructions for his care. A tracheostomy and transfer to a nursing home had been planned. His treating physicians expressed the unlikely hope of eventual improvement/

awakening and possible rehabilitation. Sue found the medical staff to be kind, yet somewhat detached and clinical. They spoke in terms of percentage chances for her father's progress and could not say with certainty whether or not he would improve.

After I spoke with her, Sue and her mother went back to the doctors and asked them to leave the clinical analysis to the side and to speak candidly, to go with their gut. This opened new horizons, since doctors often feel compelled to practice medicine with liability in mind. We are asked about probabilities and "medical certainty." This can make for defensive legalistic interactions between doctors and families. We are trained to treat, rather than to back off, especially in murky situations. Sue asked the hospitalist, Dr. Simmons Thomas, what he would do if this were his father. His demeanor changed, and to her astonishment, he teared up as he related that this was the very situation he and his family had faced only three weeks earlier. They chose to withdraw care and allow his father to die. Dr. Thomas understood, firsthand, how difficult this decision was to make and how profound an experience it was to bear witness to a parent's death.

In that moment, Sue and her mother made a vital connection with her father's physician. They became allies and accepted his advice. Dr. Thomas became comfortable enough to let down his guard and provide the best guidance he could, given the circumstances. They asked him to tell them when it was time to let go and withdraw the ventilator. They were able, as a team, to give up on heroic interventions and life supported by machines. Sue's parents had already spoken at length about spirituality, death, and what they wanted at the end of their lives. They had a living will in place. This helped the family to ease toward withdrawing treatment and allowing Larry to die without a prolonged decline in which he would have no say.

Sue showed great courage when she initiated the conversation about withdrawing treatment. Her questions and willingness to face painful truths led to a compassionate consensus among the medical team and her family members. The dialogue got everyone on the same page. If that had not happened, it is possible that Larry would have received a tracheostomy and a feeding tube and been transferred to a nursing home, only to die there at a later date. In the absence of an empathetic connection, there is a danger of medicalizing death and applying legal standards of certainty, which we as physicians frequently lack. Perhaps it is better to be guided by more nebulous standards of comfort and compassion, even if this means letting go of the ability to predict an outcome with "medical certainty." Families will sometimes cling to the chance of recovery and are willing to go the route of tracheostomy, feeding tube, and nursing home placement so as not to extinguish the possibility, no matter how unlikely, of recovery. Yet when we as physicians are faced with end-of-life decisions for our own family members, as was the case in both my and Dr. Magrinat's experience, most of us choose not to intervene, or to intervene in more limited ways and to forgo additional treatments. This allows us to celebrate the life that has been lived, rather than to focus on medical interventions.

This situation was illustrated with great clarity by the experiences of two good friends, Sue and Bill Chandler. Dr. Chandler, a neurosurgeon, was one of my professors in Ann Arbor. He retired after a heart attack, then moved with his wife, Sue, to Greensboro, to be with their son, his wife, and their two daughters. Their son and daughter-in-law are both physicians and work in our local hospital. Sue and Bill read an earlier draft of this book and gave constructive suggestions for improvements. Bill later told me that reading this book together helped them both confront their own mortality and prepare for Sue's sudden and daunting illness.

Sue and Bill were active and in excellent health. Two years ago, she began to experience painless abdominal bloating. A CT scan was obtained, which showed widely metastatic pancreatic cancer. This diagnosis carried an average life expectancy of six months. Initially, Sue didn't want any treatment. Then, she agreed to chemotherapy, but on a limited basis and only if the follow-up CT scan showed improvement. This was initiated in Ann Arbor, but they transferred her care to Greensboro to be closer to their son and grandchildren.

Sue and Bill made every decision through a filter of maintaining quality of life. They understood the implications of these choices; they had lived through Bill's experiences as a neurosurgeon, of making life-and-death decisions on a daily basis. We had tea together shortly before Sue died. She showed Kathryn and me a photograph of herself standing on the stage with her granddaughter, celebrating her victory in a dance competition. Sue cried tears of joy as she told us about this event.

A few days later, Sue had a stroke. This was likely the result of increased clotting that frequently accompanies a diagnosis of cancer. She lost the power to speak or to move the right side of her body. I met Sue, Bill, and their son Jesse (an orthopedic surgeon) in the Emergency Room to help decide on a treatment plan. Bill, who spent his career as a vascular neurosurgeon, decided which interventions to pursue and when it was time to stop. He allowed for a clot retrieval procedure to be performed and, for a while, Sue improved. But the clot recurred and her stroke symptoms of paralysis and aphasia (loss of speech) returned. At that point, they decided to move Sue to hospice and she died a few days later, five months after she was diagnosed with pancreatic cancer.

The family's experience, while marked with sadness and loss, was one of profound gratitude. They found the medical staff at every turn to be compassionate and caring. Sue, who faced her diagnosis bravely, lived as fully as she could. She said her goodbyes and celebrated with her granddaughter. In an email she sent me soon after her diagnosis, Sue told me, "I cleaned out my closets." This was something she wanted to do for herself and for her family. The family's intimate understanding of the power, and also of the shortcomings, of medical treatments allowed them to make selective use of the options available to them, while always focused on comfort, quality of life, and compassionate connections with each other.

Support groups for patients and their families exist in many healthcare institutions, but there are none for doctors. I was recently on a panel discussing end-of-life care and was struck by a story told by a nurse at our cancer center. She recalled how staff members were speaking about patients and their deaths from cancer, when Dr. Bronfman, an oncologist who always seemed taciturn and clinical, began to weep. He was overcome with sadness over the losses he had endured, of countless patients he had cared for and cared about yet was powerless to save. Dr. Bronfman had never been in a position to express his grief. There was always another patient to see, always another tragic story to contend with.

The physician is meant to be the expert, the rock, unflappable in the face of adversity or disaster. Yet one day, we become patients, too. We die just like everyone else. Try as we might, we are powerless to change any of that. In the end, a sympathetic word, a hug, released a torrent of emotion for this devoted, successful oncologist. With my sister's death, I feel this suppressed ache; I wish I had been able to save her. When I look back on my career, how is my sister's case any different from those of my other patients? True, I was more personally invested, but her life was no more significant or meaningful than the lives of my other patients, except to me.

"I don't know" is not typically part of a neurosurgeon's vocabulary. Yet, honest connection with patients requires the ability to express doubt. Medical delivery is not generally set up for this. Patients want to believe in the authoritative offerings of modern medicine, and doctors want to believe in their ability to heal and help their patients. Both want success and shrink from failure. Neither is comfortable when things don't work or do not go according to plan.

Currently, approximately 55 percent of physicians admit to being burned out. This burnout ranges from job dissatisfaction all the way to the decision to take early retirement and can manifest in their lives as substance abuse, divorce, and even suicide, depending on the severity of this experience. As Stacy Wentworth indicated in her interview, we are poorly trained to handle the implications of death or failure. We have a lot on our plates, so at times counseling patients about death and dying feels like yet another burden. As physicians, we are expected to solve problems and to work, often it seems, without stop. These responsibilities are in addition to growing dissatisfaction with electronic medical records, regular arguments with insurance companies, and medicolegal aspects of practice.

Death and dying contribute to physician burnout. This includes "compassion fatigue," or the feeling of being overwhelmed by regular and seemingly unrelenting loss, and also our inability to process grief and loss personally and within our professional lives. If we look, there are solutions readily at hand. Generally, in patient care, we have been transitioning from being isolated practitioners to becoming members of treatment teams, in which patient care duties are shared with others. The care of dying patients should be no different.

The patient's experience, both in and out of hospitals, needs to be designed with compassion as the primary driver of care decisions and environments, allowing patients to best meet their needs. As Matt Manning said, people should not have to check their dignity at the door upon entering the ICU. Patients lose their clothes, possessions, and identities when they don a hospital gown and get hooked up to machines in a hospital bed. Research supports ways to improve the patient experience and maintain dignity in the ICU. My sister surrounded herself with large photos of her husband and children during each hospitalization. This helped her maintain her identity and reminded her that she was more than a patient. Staff and visitors recognized that this was a person rooted in a world far removed from the cancer ward.

Something as simple as placing large monitors in positions of prominence on which photos of family members could be displayed would go a long way toward humanizing patients and grounding them in the lives they have been pulled away from. These would not interfere with treatment, they would not pose an infection risk, and they are inexpensive. Perhaps patients checking in for long-term care could arrive with a few possessions and a flash drive with selected photos to plug into the monitor. This might help decrease "sundowning," a common phenomenon in elderly patients who become disoriented during hospitalizations. Efforts to maintain night and day routines, respecting our circadian rhythms, would also help prevent the disorientation that comes with the sleep deprivation, which is a hallmark of a stay in the ICU.

Sound management is similarly important. For many people, music connects them with their world and often provides a calming or transporting influence. It would be simple to invite patients and their families to bring a playlist of their favorite music to listen to during their hospitalization. Particularly at the end of life, having your favorite music with you might help take the edge off the fear and help soothe the patient and family. In both instances, simple modifications to the inpatient room environment would go a long way toward improving the patient's experience.

While I visited Victoria, I was struck by the disruption caused by the frequent beeping of IV pumps. My sister would hear a beep, then summon a nurse, who would come into her room, often after many minutes, to address the source of the alarm. Yet alarms do not prioritize the severity of a problem and can frighten the patient. This could all be done more effectively through wireless communication to the nurse, without the intermediate step of the patient being "alarmed," only to report the problem to the nurse, who has to come check the pump, identify the source of the problem, turn off the alarm, often leave the room to get a new IV bag, and then return with the new medication. This would cut out two steps, response times could be monitored, and the patient would not be disturbed or awakened. Here, technologies could be adopted to improve the patient's experience and replace intrusive alarms that currently disrupt patients.

New technologies need to improve rather than detract from patients' experiences. Health systems need to implement these technologies with empathy in mind. There are many ways technology interferes with connecting practitioners with their patients, but this often seems less a failure inherent in the technology itself and more often is our failure for allowing this to happen. We have let electronic medical record systems intrude on and erode doctor-patient interactions; the necessity of making computer keystrokes has supplanted nurse-patient connections. Yet, this does not need to be the case. Technology needs to be implemented with the core values of patients (autonomy, respect, experience) in mind, rather than relegating these to an afterthought. Thus, photo displays, sound systems, and wireless IV pump notifications that do away with ever-present "beeps" are simple technological innovations that would go a long way toward improving and humanizing patients' hospital stays.

By illustration of poorly implemented technologies, my father-in-law, Gary Crawley, who is being treated for multiple myeloma (a blood cancer), described his ongoing experience with check-in at two cancer centers. The first involves a detailed review of his personal and insurance information with multiple repetitive questions every time he arrives for treatment, no matter how frequently his appointments occur, despite the fact that nothing in his personal profile has changed. He finds this process dehumanizing, time-consuming, and irritating.

At the second cancer center, he presents his identification card to the clerk who greets him warmly, swipes it in the computer, asks if anything has changed, to which he replies "No," then takes a seat. Check-in at this center is easy, while at the other one it is burdensome. This is not a problem with the technology itself, but instead reflects the way the staff has been instructed to gather and verify patient information and interact with hospital information systems. The two different health systems send a clear message to patients about how they are valued well before any actual care has commenced. At the first, the act of obtaining information has mistakenly been valued higher than an empathetic greeting of the patient, while at the second, the patient's comfort and convenience is more highly valued. Ironically, I suspect the quality of information gathered in both centers is identical.

Other disruptive influences include the shift-work model in hospitals, which does not respect the natural cycle of day and night and is not conducive to healing. When I am in the hospital in the middle of the night, I am frequently surprised by the level of noise surrounding me. Staff members confer in the hallways and nursing stations, carts crash and bang, and alarms beep, chirp, and wail all through the night. Noise levels in the ICU can rise to 85 dB at night (the sound of a food blender running), whereas 35 dB would be more appropriate for maintaining a restful environment. Why are we surprised when patients gradually wear down with exhaustion during prolonged hospitalizations and become confused or, at times, delirious?

Part of the dehumanizing process of a hospitalization is the imposition of "medically indicated" routines that are performed for the convenience of the hospital personnel rather than out of regard for the patients. This includes waking patients up in the middle of the night for routine vital sign monitoring and imposing schedules on activities that could be allowed to be more spontaneous without any detriment to the quality of care. It would be wonderful for hospitals to begin to consider patient comfort as a high priority, rather than focusing on task completion according to a rigid external schedule. While patients need twenty-four-hour monitoring and shift work is an inherent feature of hospital staffing, far more could be done to respect patient needs and sleep-wake cycles.

Mary Magrinat's experience resonated with me. She had an intravenous port placed surgically for the administration of chemotherapy. The doctor placed it "for the convenience of the nurses," so that it would be easy to access. The trade-off for Mary was an unsightly and readily visible port that she was unable to hide without buying new, higher-cut clothing. She resented this, as it was uncomfortable and served as a constant reminder to everyone around her that she was ill. Eventually, Mary insisted the port be removed. Whenever possible, we should think about what is best for the patient and make decisions according to those standards, rather than what is convenient for the medical staff. Many things are done in hospitals and medical practice out of tradition and/ or in the name of efficiency. It is time we turn this way of thinking on its head and reshape medical-care delivery so that it is based on the needs and respect of the patients we are charged to serve.

Healthcare will improve if physicians and medical systems develop greater empathy for patients and for each other. I have given a few examples of how to redesign care delivery and patient care environments. There are many more ways patient care could (and should) be redesigned. Physicians, also, must give voice to their experiences, many of which have shaped their personal and professional lives. Doing so would benefit practitioners, the health systems they work for, and the patients they serve. I encourage medical schools and health systems to support the creation and implementation of courses and workshops, which could combine readings, empathy training, and interview training, in which physicians are encouraged to share some of their experiences with each other.

These concerns are now more widely recognized than when I was trained as a physician and later as a neurosurgeon. Medical schools are teaching the importance of patient respect and compassion, and surgical training programs are also changing; cultures of abuse are disappearing, as are the legendary professors known for their towering egos and harsh didactic manners. A surgeon's bad behavior could once be excused by the perception of his daring and surgical competence. In the face of data indicating that a lack of compassion and connection with patients leads to poorer surgical outcomes and compromised patient safety, it is clearly time to end these practices and shift the surgical culture to one in which compassion has a central place in every operating room and surgeons are encouraged to acknowledge their emotions, rather than to repress them. The same is true for hospitals and healthcare as a whole. It is time for us to put patients, rather than diseases, at the center.

compassion and coronavirus

What is most impressive in the hospitals is not the ventilators, CT scanners or other high-tech wizardry. It's the compassion and courage of health workers, and the intervention that struck me the most was decidedly low-tech—the hand-holding. —NICHOLAS KRISTOF, "LIFE AND DEATH IN THE 'HOT ZONE'"*

Each time I thought I was done writing this book, an event occurred that caused me to rethink everything. The first was the night Pat had his hemorrhage in LA, ushering in his death. The second, which developed as my agent Linda shopped my book proposal to publishers, was the gradually unrolling coronavirus pandemic. Over the course of spring 2020, we watched as the infection swept across the world. Life as we knew it stopped. Jobs and businesses disappeared; people were quarantined and became ill. Everyone's life has been profoundly altered by effects ranging from job loss, hunger, social isolation, illness, and death.

For the first time in my lifetime, a sense of grief and loss has washed over the entire planet. Certainly, these are experiences we each have individually: they define the human condition. Yet, during the pandemic, this has been an experience we have all shared. It has etched itself into our collective psyche; we will be forever changed because of it. As I said to a dear friend on the accidental death of his teenage son, who died at the height of the pandemic: grief connects us with our better selves. There's no going back.

That said, I wouldn't wish it on anyone. The losses we have felt during this time have been magnified in their intensity, as the rituals we rely on to mark the transitions of our lives have been disallowed. My friend's family was unable to have a funeral for his son, just as others have died alone and been summarily buried without celebration. Weddings and graduations have been canceled, births and deaths have been unattended. In the periods of both Victoria's and Pat's deaths, being present and surrounded by family members had great power, gathering to eat together to make decisions was restorative, and having the opportunity to reminisce and attend their funerals helped provide a path toward healing.

Practicing medicine through the pandemic, we wear masks on setting foot in the hospital. Patients are kept in their rooms without family members. The surgical waiting room is emptied and the only contact we have with patients' families is by telephone. Simple yet meaningful gestures, like a touch or a smile, are curtailed. Physical contact no longer conveys connection; instead it carries fear and the possibility of infection. It is very difficult to establish empathetic connections when everyone is covered with masks or, in more extreme situations, by masks, goggles, and face shields.

I watch as my elderly parents isolate themselves to prevent infection. We cut off visitation to my father-in-law, already immunocompromised from chemotherapy for blood cancer, for fear of exposure to the coronavirus, even though he lives down the street from us. This makes sense, since I was likely to become exposed. My father, in his early nineties, sees people only incidentally while he shops for groceries every few weeks. Otherwise, he is completely alone. His only contact with his family is through video chats.

What's so different now? For a start, we are all on a level playing field. This is a new virus, so we are all learning about treating it, together. Physicians are no longer in a position of power with asymmetric information. Patients are the ones who usually feel openly vulnerable and afraid. Doctors typically try to cover that up. If anything, now it's the opposite. The doctors are at greater risk than the general population, since sick patients are concentrated in hospitals and no one has any protection from the virus, other than by avoiding it. In fact, a tension exists between healthcare workers and those who aren't in healthcare. Social isolation is currently the only way to prevent viral spread and to protect healthcare workers, at least until there is greater testing, contact tracing, better treatments, or a vaccine. In the meantime, physicians are dependent on everyone else for their own protection. Thus, the tables are turned. Patients and society now have the upper hand. It is the physicians who are now vulnerable.

I was recently exposed to a patient with COVID-19. She came into the ER with a large subdural hemorrhage, from which she was dying. She had a blown pupil (a sign of impending herniation and death), was no longer moving one side of her body, and was rapidly losing consciousness. We intubated her emergently and rushed her off to surgery. The pharmacist corrected her blood clotting disorder. Routine questions of her husband raised our suspicions when he said she had been coughing for the last few days and had a low-grade fever, even though her temperature in the ER was normal. We took precautions in surgery and everyone wore protective gear, including N95 masks.

After her surgery, we tested our patient (our hospital had only recently attained the ability to perform rapid testing with a two-hour turnaround). Her test came back positive. We moved her from the Neuro-ICU to the newly created COVID-ICU. Testing allowed us to screen patients and protect ourselves from inadvertent exposure. Without it, many healthcare workers would have been exposed, potentially sickened, and died. By my estimation, almost thirty people had cared for this patient, including EMS, nursing, physicians, transporters, OR personnel, housekeeping, respiratory therapists, and radiation technologists. Once we knew she was infected, we were able to take precautions and wear appropriate personal protective equipment (PPE). But some of us had been exposed.

A lack of preparation for the pandemic, including testing, ventilators, and PPE, has intensified the anxieties of physicians and healthcare workers. So, too, has the slow acceptance of social distancing measures—the incomplete adherence to or downright rejection of these simple interventions. Instead of relying on proven public health and scientifically based measures to prevent disease spread in the US, political manipulation, disinformation, bribery, and greed have been allowed to dictate social policy, all at the expense of the safety of the general population and of healthcare workers in particular. There has been a pervasive leadership vacuum and a lack of will to harness widespread energy and goodwill for the greater good.

Yet, despite these failings, something extraordinary has happened. The unflinching bravery, generosity, and self-sacrifice of my fellow healthcare workers as they continue to look after their patients, even while exposing themselves and their families to risk, inspires me. In the middle ages, doctors were some of the first to leave infected areas at the outset of the bubonic plague. Here, we have met the challenge head on.

After my initial fear at being exposed to COVID-19, I went into the COVID-ICU to see how my patient was doing. I have to admit I was extremely frightened. I didn't know what I would find there. As I stood outside the locked doors to the ICU and hit the button to activate the intercom and camera, I wasn't sure what to expect. A young nurse came to the door and escorted me in. Another nurse showed me how to don PPE. I was already wearing an N95 mask with a Level 1 mask over the top of it. I gelled my hands, then put on a plastic gown, gloves, and a face shield over my glasses. I gelled the outside of my gloves, then slid open the door to the patient's room, past the IV pumps parked in front of her door, within easy reach of the medical team, so that they could be accessed remotely. Her nurse accompanied me into the room. We slid the door closed behind us.

My patient was sitting up in bed. She was awake and answered my questions. She had no recollection of what had happened to her or of how close she had come to dying. Her pupil had come back down to normal size, although her eyelid continued to droop, but she was moving her arms and legs well with no signs of paralysis. I removed the drain I placed in her head at the time of her surgery and sealed the hole in her scalp with some staples. This would allow her to get up and walk with the physical therapists.

We threw the drain and stapler into a trash receptacle, gelled our hands again, then carefully removed the PPE and disposed of the gown and gloves in the trash, while keeping the facemask and N95 mask to be sterilized for reuse.

My patient continued to recover and soon after, she was discharged home, to continue her convalescence with her husband. Further questioning revealed that he had likely had COVID-19 before his wife and was now fully recovered. He was an essential manufacturing worker who was helping produce personal care items during the pandemic. We planned for her to come back to the office to have her staples removed in a month. This would allow her time to recover and hopefully to no longer be infectious. Not only did she not die as I initially feared, she went on to make a full recovery.

She came back to my office with her husband several weeks after her surgery. COVID had caused her to develop a coagulopathy (her blood became too thin) and she had spontaneously hemorrhaged, developing a near-fatal subdural hematoma (blood on the outside of her brain). By the time she returned, she had recovered from her COVID infection. Her blood-clotting disorder had also resolved and she had no lingering impairment from her near fatal hemorrhage. Her husband sat with her and filled in the details of her illness, since before that moment, I had only spoken with him on the phone and had never met him in person.

My patient is a lovely person who had worked as a high school guidance counselor for the last thirty years. The couple were extraordinarily grateful for the care they had received and I took a photograph of her with her thumbs up, seated next to her husband, both in facemasks. I sent the photo to the ER team and pharmacist who initially saved her life, to the Neuro-ICU team, to the OR team, to the COVID-ICU team, and to the CEO and CMO of the hospital. They had all played a vital role in saving this woman's life. We all worked together on her behalf. Each of us understood the risks inherent in our jobs and did them anyway. A husband and wife, who seemed to me to be very much in love, narrowly avoided a horrific loss and will survive intact.

The staff in the COVID-ICU was inspiring. They all volunteered to work there, accepting the risks of exposure. They were kind to each other and to their patients. They were reassuring to me, as they watched me don and doff the PPE and supervised my every movement to make sure I didn't breach any of the protocols designed to protect us from inadvertent exposure to the virus. The doctors and nurses were brave. They were calm and deliberate. The entire unit was suffused with a spirit of compassion. The very things I have been advocating for in this book were on display. There was a shared sense of purpose, a feeling of resolute determination, and no longer a disconnection between patients and their caregivers. They were all on the same page, all fighting and afraid of the same thing, each at risk of infection, and of dying.

For everyone's safety, family members were excluded from the ICU. But rather than fostering indifference, this seemed to engender greater consideration. The staff went out of their way to connect patients and their family members. They reported changes in condition and regularly updated concerned family members. My patient's nurse went back into her room after I left to help her FaceTime her husband. While I went in with trepidation, I left inspired by and proud of my fellow healthcare workers.

That same evening, my neighbors gathered in the street to say thanks to "the COVID-19 warriors." They banged pots, tapped bottles, sang, and beat makeshift drums made from trashcans. They were celebrating the sacrifices made, and the risks taken, by the healthcare workers who went toward, rather than away from, danger.

This common purpose, shared vulnerability, and tremendous courage in the face of danger has been seen the world over. Medical personnel have volunteered and gone to New York to help at the heart of the pandemic, risking their own lives and, less directly, the lives of their families. They have done the same in Italy. What I saw frightened me, yet this pales in comparison to what healthcare workers have had to face in the Bronx or other besieged communities. There has been a general, and heartwarming, willingness to face personal danger for a greater good. Since there is no available treatment or cure for the virus, the willingness to face the pandemic head-on exposes practitioners directly to dangers they can try to minimize but can in no way control. The threat is very real; witness the number of healthcare workers who have died from the coronavirus.

Unlike with my sister or Pat's diagnoses and treatment, everyone who comes in contact with the virus faces, with the caveat of comorbidities, the same relative risk. Yes, the healthcare workers understand details of patient care that the general population doesn't possess. That is why they are useful. But, in reality, this affords them little to no protection from harm. The distinction between patient and doctor is less clear. They now have shared vulnerability and risk. The knowledge and power differentials have been flattened. A willingness to go into harm's way is, at its core, an act of compassion.

The backdrop of political anti-lockdown protests, claims of "hoax," and rejection of science and public health measures are a distraction from what I have witnessed in caring for patients during the pandemic. The greater message has been one of humanity and compassion, of people supporting each other, and of coming together. We have experienced an event of far-reaching historical significance collectively. Most of us, particularly those of us in healthcare, have dug into ourselves and risen to the occasion, going beyond our comfort zones to help others in need. My neighbor, a retired periodontist, volunteered on a farm to help harvest crops and then took them to a food bank to distribute to the hungry. A local restauranteur, Reto Biaggi, in an effort to keep his business afloat but also to spread goodwill, kindness, and support within his community, has been providing takeaway meals at inexpensive prices for anyone who places an order. He and his staff are using scrupulous technique and food handling, with masks and gloves. They bring the sealed meals out to the customer's car and are giving away desserts to healthcare workers as a way of expressing their thanks.

These approaches are relevant to the message I have been trying to relay throughout this book. Some have adopted a defended, self-preserving posture, while others have recognized that a radically new situation demands innovative approaches. These have required us to apply adaptability, resilience, courage, compassion, and love. How we confront external threats is not dissimilar to how we must face the disruption of a difficult disease diagnosis or the mortal illness of a family member. Once this has occurred, things are forever different. We can use the skills we have at our disposal to adjust to this new reality, but we can't wish it away or pretend it isn't happening. Will we be flexible and adaptive, or dig our heels in and refuse to budge? Will we cling to old truths and deny new realities out of fear or will we admit what we don't know and can't control and embrace this fear and uncertainty as a necessary fact of our lives? Will we see each other for who we are or dwell in shadows and projections of our own making?

My experience with my patient with COVID-19 and the subdural hemorrhage is not unlike the experiences I had with my sister and her husband, in that it forced me out of my normal level of comfort and familiarity into a challenging situation, which caused me fear and stress. My willingness to face these challenges was emblematic of the emotional agility I am advocating that we embrace: I was forced to confront my fear without retreating from it, to summon courage and go into the COVID-ICU and to care for my patient who I knew was infected. My fear was of the unknown; an anxiety that I might get infected or that I would inadvertently harm my family members by exposing them to coronavirus infection. None of this happened. Instead, I have grown as a human being and as a doctor. I saved a life. I was working with inspiring, courageous, generous, and selfless people who were, themselves, willing to face their fears, give of themselves, and take on risk. And look what we are able to do as a result! Together, as healthcare professionals, we must hold our heads high and allow ourselves to feel pride in what we have accomplished.

Moving toward greater compassion is ultimately the most fulfilling path we can take. Making health systems more patient-focused and friendly, meeting patients where they are, inviting them to express their greatest concerns and fears, incorporating their life circumstances into decisions, flattening the power and knowledge differentials between practitioner and patient, and striving for humanity and compassion as the basis for the healthcare environments and our decision-making must be our objective. The Healing Garden is an example of harnessing the power of grief and loss for a greater good. While this comes out of the anguish of personal loss, it provides a gift to others for their own healing, as well as a shift toward a more holistic and nurturing approach to patient care.

The more I strive toward empathy and compassion in the care I render, the more I see what we need to change and improve. Like an itch you can't stop scratching, the piercing losses I experienced have opened my eyes and made me reach for these goals, surrounding myself with like-minded people who look at systems as having the potential for improvement and change, partnering with others across disciplines, like palliative care and nursing, who have much to add as we strive to humanize and elevate the care we provide for our patients. As we have learned in this pandemic, it is not "me" and "you," only "us."

At the same time as healthcare workers are showing compassion for others while exposing ourselves to risk, we are also having to contend with grief and loss. So many of us have lost so much: lives of family members and friends, jobs and the rhythms of our lives, the social connections that bind us together. In the space of three months, I watched as my daughter's senior year in college came to a sudden halt, no farewells and closure, her graduation canceled. She had job plans for the coming year, now on hold. Our middle son was in the midst of applying to medical school and starting a new job. These things were also delayed. The world over, situations like these are commonplace, with job losses, business collapses, death, and dislocation.

How do we find the resilience to overcome these misfortunes? How can we use our heartache to channel our energies toward productive engagement, rather than defeat, isolation, or selfishness? How can we use these losses to bring clarity and focus to our efforts? We must fight to maintain our humanity, to bolster ourselves, to come together and support each other. There clearly are limits to resilience. Witness the death, by suicide, of Dr. Lorna M. Breen. She was a frontline emergency department doctor at New York Presbyterian Allen Hospital, caring for an onslaught of COVID-19 patients "who were dying before they could even be taken out of ambulances." At some point, there can be too much sorrow, too much loss, a numbing, seemingly endless procession of the dead and dying. Although I did not know Dr. Breen, I worry that she might have been overwhelmed by feelings of sadness and despair, perhaps by a sense that she had failed to save patients, who in reality were unsalvageable. It is hard, as a physician, to feel that society does not support your efforts to treat and save patients; we have provided insufficient PPE and also increased case counts by retreating prematurely from social distancing. It seems unfair to expect so much from a few, while not supporting, protecting, or valuing their contributions toward our general welfare.

Honoring healthcare workers as heroes doesn't obviate the expectation that we all support and protect each other. What good is a yard sign celebrating "COVID warriors" if you are unwilling to wear a mask to protect others (including healthcare workers) more vulnerable than yourself? Since wearing a mask protects others from you, but not necessarily you from others in terms of viral transmission, two conclusions follow: The first is that this is an essential gesture of mutual respect, which only makes sense if we all adhere to the same social standards, ideally driven by science and leadership, striving to curtail the pandemic. The second is that mask-wearing is a true expression of empathy.

In the midst of these often crushing blows, there has been a calm and serenity that's emerged. A worldwide reset of priorities, both personal and collective, an acknowledgment of the importance of connecting with each other and the power of empathy and compassion in the way we conduct our relationships and our lives. I hope we can build on that through mutual support at both the individual and societal levels.

ACKNOWLEDGMENTS

What started as a six-month project has turned into a six-year adventure. I have discovered intersecting worlds outside of neurosurgery that I never knew existed. I am profoundly indebted to my sister Victoria and to her husband, Pat, whose stories I have had the privilege to tell and to their sons, Nick and Will, who live their legacy. I am proud of them all for their devotion to each other and grateful for their warm and loving household, frequently overflowing with the kindest friends, concerned family members, and gourmet meals. Pat trusted me to include Victoria's journals in this book. I have tried to respect her wishes and the spirit of her work, editing for grammar and eliminating repetition, as she did not have the opportunity to review her own work. Alison Larkin encouraged Victoria to write about her experiences in a journal and also urged me to write as well. Without Alison's early efforts, I doubt a book would have ever have materialized.

I am indebted to Leslie and Steve Mackler, who shared their experience with Leslie's ovarian cancer and chemotherapy. Those early conversations provided the germ for the formal interviews I conducted in the book. Each of my interviewees is extremely busy, yet each was willing to meet with me to discuss their personal experiences and to share their stories and reflections, unfiltered. Dr. Sean Fischer understood what I was hoping to learn about Victoria's care and was courageous and trusting enough to speak candidly with me after my sister's death. Similarly, Drs. Matt Manning, Stacy Wentworth, Gus Magrinat, and Irving Lugo, and my former patient William E. Williams, were unflinching in their honesty and willingness to answer my questions. So, too, were Mary Magrinat and Sally Pagliai. Mary kindly provided photographs and captions of The Healing Garden.

My wife, Kathryn, has been unbelievably supportive and a tireless and excellent editor. She was willing to put her own writing on hold to assist me with this project. Her mother, Margaret Crawley, has also been a careful editor and critic, as have my mother, Elizabeth Buchanek, and my sister, Caroline Stern. Our children, Ben, David, and Abby have also been steadfast in their encouragement. I hope that someday I will be able to return the favor.

Julie Silver's Harvard Writer's Course opened doors for me. There, I met Linda Konner, who saw value in a reimagined version of this book and agreed to become my agent. She has been a tireless advocate. Linda introduced me to Valerie Killeen at Central Recovery Press, who chose to publish *Grief Connects Us*. Nancy Schenck, from CRP, has been a wonderful editor and a joy to work with, as have Patrick Hughes, John Davis, and Marisa Jackson. Erika Heilman helped me craft the first version of my book proposal. From the world of journalism, I am grateful to Roberta Zeff of the *New York Times*, who took a chance on an unknown writer. Also, I appreciate the help of Vivian Toy and Karen Heller. M.C. Sullivan, who runs the Palliative Care program, reached out to me from the Archdiocese of Boston. Other writers have been supportive and encouraging. These include Drs. Sanjay Gupta, who graciously wrote the Foreword to this book, Michael Attas, Mikkael Sekeres, Abraham Verghese, Henry Marsh, Helen Riess, BJ Miller, Pauline Chen, and James Doty. Margaret Edson, a friend from Sidwell Friends forty years ago, graciously agreed to endorse my work.

I am grateful to my office staff, Lori Underhill, Orren Miller, Pamela Sizemore, and Robin Young. Lori and Pam transcribed the interviews and were helpful and encouraging readers. Drs. Karin Muraszko, Marlienne Goldin, Dave Joslin, Mike Sheinberg, Kyle Jackson, Bill Chandler and his wife Sue, Sue and Joe Upton, Kevin Daniels, Dr. Hans Coester and his wife Cindi, Dr. Jeffrey Segal and his wife Shelley, Jennifer Steinl, Dr. Chris Langston, Dr. Jonathan Berry, Anne and Emma Stringer, Dr. Peter Crawley and his wife Ingrid, David and Catherine Mayer, Dr. Carswell Jackson, Mack Sperling, Kimberly C. Paul, Andy and Dorothy Winkler, and Brian Poteat, R.N. were also supportive friends and discerning readers. Laura Simon Klein encouraged me to write for the *New York Times*. Members of the Cone Health medical staff, including Drs. Bruce Swords, Mary Jo Cagle, Pat Wright, Jay Wyatt, and William Morgan, along with Joan Evans, Angela Marsh, Jami Goldberg, Mickey Foster, Ann Marie Madden, Cynthia Rizzo, Robert Hickling, and Terry Akin were helpful readers and mentors. Margaret Wynn did a heroic job as a reference librarian, both tirelessly searching the medical literature and assembling references. I found inspiration and support from Dr. Sarah Soule and Dr. Abraham Verghese, who run a wonderful course at Stanford University, The Innovative Health Care Leader, which I had the privilege to attend. Abraham connected me with Irene Connelly, who has been a phenomenal editor. Patient, sensitive, gifted, and insightful, she brought out the best of this work. Without Irene's help, this book would never have seen the light of day.

Finally, I am appreciative of my partners and staff at Carolina Neurosurgery and Spine Associates (CNSA) and of the patients who trust us with their medical care. We strive to deliver the best possible neurosurgical care for our patients each and every day.

REFERENCES

part one

CHAPTER ONE: DIAGNOSIS

"Acute myeloid leukemia." MedlinePlus. Accessed February 20, 2017. https://medlineplus.gov/acutemyeloidleukemia.html.

"Adult acute myeloid leukemia treatment (PDQ®)—Health professional version." NIH National Cancer Institute. 2017. https://www.cancer.gov/types/leukemia/hp/adult-aml-treatment-pdq.

"Adult acute myeloid leukemia treatment (PDQ®)—Patient version." NIH National Cancer Institute. 2017. https://www.cancer.gov/types/leukemia/patient/adult-aml-treatment-pdq.

Harry, B. *The Paul McCartney Encyclopedia*. London: Virgin, 2002.

CHAPTER TWO: LEARNING TO TIE KNOTS/ ARC OF A CAREER

Ferrara, Felicetto and Charles A Schiffer. "Acute Myeloid Leukaemia in Adults." *The Lancet* 381, no. 9865 (2013): 484–95. https://doi.org/10.1016/s0140-6736(12)61727-9.

Quintás-Cardama, Alfonso, and Jorge E. Cortes. "Chronic Myeloid Leukemia: Diagnosis and Treatment." *Mayo Clinic Proceedings* 81, no. 7 (2006): 973–88. https://doi.org/10.4065/81.7.973.

Singer, Robert J., Christopher S. Ogilvy, and Guy Rordorf. (2016) "Screening for intracranial aneurysm." In J. Biller (Ed.), *UpToDate*, 2016. https://www.uptodate.com/contents/screening-for-intracranial-aneurysm.

part two

CHAPTER THREE: THE PATIENT'S PERSPECTIVE

Halt the development of malignancies:

Zilfou, J. T. and S. W. Lowe. "Tumor Suppressive Functions of p53." *Cold Spring Harbor Perspectives in Biology* 1, no. 5 (2009). https://doi.org/10.1101/cshperspect.a001883.

Propensity to developing leukemia:

Tomasetti, C., L. Li, and B. Vogelstein. (2017). "Stem cell divisions, somatic mutations, cancer etiology, and cancer prevention." *Science*, 355(6331), 1330–34. https://doi.org/10.1126/science.aaf9011.

ADDITIONAL SOURCES

"Adult acute myeloid leukemia treatment (PDQ®)—patient version." NIH National Cancer Institute. (2017). https://www.cancer.gov/types/leukemia/patient/adult-aml-treatment-pdq.

"Bone marrow (stem cell) donation." MedlinePlus. August 15, 2016. https://medlineplus.gov/ency/patientinstructions/000839.htm.

"BRCA1 & BRCA2: Cancer risk and genetic testing." NIH National Cancer Institute. (2015). https://www.cancer.gov/about-cancer/causes-prevention/genetics/brca-fact-sheet.

Desouza, R. M., H. Shaweis, C. Han, V. Sivasubramiam, L. Brazil, R. Beaney, G. Sadler, S. Al-Sarraj, T. Hampton, and J. Logan. "Has the Survival of Patients with Glioblastoma Changed over the Years?" *British Journal of Cancer* 114, no. 2 (2015): 146–50. https://doi.org/10.1038/bjc.2015.421.

"Donate bone marrow." Be the Match. April 22, 2016. https://bethematch.org/support-the-cause/donate-bone-marrow/.

"Donor resources." Gift of Life. Accessed February 22, 2017. https://www.giftoflife.org/page/content/donorresources.

"Epigenomics (Fact Sheet)." National Human Genome Research Institute. (2016). https://www.genome.gov/27532724/Epigenomics-Fact-Sheet.

"Facts about Neupogen® (Filgrastim)." Centers for Disease Control and Prevention. April 16, 2016. https://emergency.cdc.gov/radiation/neupogenfacts.asp.

"Filgrastim, Filgrastim-sndz, Tbo-filgrastim Injection: MedlinePlus drug information." MedlinePlus. February 7, 2017. https://medlineplus.gov/druginfo/meds/a692033.html.

"Genetic counseling for hereditary breast and ovarian cancer." Centers for Disease Control and Prevention. (2014). https://www.cdc.gov/genomics/resources/diseases/breast_ovarian_cancer/counseling.htm.

"Glioblastoma (GBM)." American Brain Tumor Association. (2014). http://www.abta.org/brain-tumor-information/types-of-tumors/glioblastoma.html.

"High-dose chemotherapy and stem cell transplant for acute lymphocytic leukemia." American Cancer Society. Accessed February 22, 2017. https://www.cancer.org/cancer/acute-lymphocytic-leukemia/treating/bone-marrow-stem-cell.html.

Mayo Clinic staff. "Blood and bone marrow donation." May 30, 2014. http://www.mayoclinic.org/tests-procedures/bone-marrow/basics/definition/PRC-20020055?p=1.

Mirimanoff, René-Olivier, Thierry Gorlia, Warren Mason, Martin J. Van Den Bent, Rolf-Dieter Kortmann, Barbara Fisher, Michele Reni, Alba A. Brandes, Jüergen Curschmann, Salvador Villa, et al. "Radiotherapy and Temozolomide for Newly Diagnosed Glioblastoma: Recursive Partitioning Analysis of the EORTC 26981/22981-NCIC CE3 Phase III Randomized Trial." *Journal of Clinical Oncology* 24, no. 16 (2006): 2563–69. https://doi.org/10.1200/jco.2005.04.5963.

Neergaard, Lauran. "Science says: Who and what is to blame for cancer?" *U.S. News and World Report.* March 23, 2017. https://www.usnews.com/news/news/articles/2017-03-23/science-says-who-and-what-is-to-blame-for-cancer.

Park, John K., Tiffany Hodges, Leopold Arko, Michael Shen, Donna Dello Iacono, Adrian Mcnabb, Nancy Olsen Bailey, Teri Nguyen Kreisl, Fabio M. Iwamoto, Joohee Sul, et al. "Scale to Predict Survival after Surgery for Recurrent Glioblastoma Multiforme." *Journal of Clinical Oncology* 28, no. 24 (2010): 3838–43. https://doi.org/10.1200/jco.2010.30.0582.

Polivka, Jiri Jr., Jiri Polivka, Lubos Holubec, Tereza Kubikova, Vladimir Priban, Ondrej Hes, Kristyna Pivovarcikova, and Inka Treskova. "Advances in experimental targeted therapy and immunotherapy for patients with glioblastoma multiforme." *Anticancer Research,* 37, no 1 (2017): 21–33. https://doi.org/10.21873/anticanres.11285.

Ray, Surabh, Machaon M. Bonafede, and Nimish A. Mohile. "Treatment patterns, survival, and healthcare costs of patients with malignant gliomas in a large US commercially insured population." *American Health & Drug Benefits,* 7, no 3 (2014): 140–49.

Scott, Jacob G., Luc Bauchet, Tyler J. Fraum, Lakshmi Nayak, Anna R. Cooper, Samuel T. Chao, John H. Suh, Michael A. Vogelbaum, David M. Peereboom, Sonia Zouaoui, et al. "Recursive Partitioning Analysis of Prognostic Factors for Glioblastoma Patients Aged 70 Years or Older." *Cancer* 118, no. 22 (2012): 5595–5600. https://doi.org/10.1002/cncr.27570.

Sekeres, Mikkael. *When Blood Breaks Down: Life Lessons From Leukemia*. Boston, MA: MIT Press, 2020.

Shah, Binay Kumar, Amir Bista, and Sandhya Sharma. "Survival Trends in Elderly Patients with Glioblastoma in the United States: a Population-Based Study." *Anticancer Research* 36, no. 9 (2016): 4883–86. https://doi.org/10.21873/anticanres.11052.

"Stem cell transplant for acute myeloid leukemia." American Cancer Society. Accessed February 22, 2017. https://www.cancer.org/cancer/acute-myeloid-leukemia/treating/bone-marrow-stem-cell-transplant.html.

Stone, J. "What you need to know on world bone marrow day." *Forbes*. September 18, 2015. http://www.forbes.com/sites/judystone/2015/09/18/world-bone-marrow-donor-day-give-the-gift-of-life/.

Stupp, Roger, Monika E. Hegi, Warren P Mason, Martin J. Van Den Bent, Martin J B Taphoorn, Robert C. Janzer, Samuel K. Ludwin, Anouk Allgeier, Barbara Fisher, Karl Belanger, et al. "Effects of Radiotherapy with Concomitant and Adjuvant Temozolomide versus Radiotherapy Alone on Survival in Glioblastoma in a Randomised Phase III Study: 5-Year Analysis of the EORTC-NCIC Trial." *The Lancet Oncology* 10, no. 5 (2009): 459–66. https://doi.org/10.1016/s1470-2045(09)70025-7.

"Temozolomide injection." MedlinePlus. February 15, 2013. https://medlineplus.gov/druginfo/meds/a613002.html.

"Temozolomide oral." Medline Plus. January 15, 2016. https://medlineplus.gov/druginfo/meds/a601250.html.

Tomasetti, Cristian, Lu Li, and Bert Vogelstein. "Stem Cell Divisions, Somatic Mutations, Cancer Etiology, and Cancer Prevention." *Science* 355, no. 6331 (2017): 1330–34. https://doi.org/10.1126/science.aaf9011.

Zilfou, J. T. and S. W. Lowe. "Tumor Suppressive Functions of p53." Cold Spring Harbor Perspectives in Biology 1, no. 5 (2009). https://doi.org/10.1101/cshperspect.a001883.

CHAPTER FOUR: RECONNECTING/FIRST VISIT

Groopman, Jerome. "The Transformation: Is it possible to control cancer without killing it?" *The New Yorker*. September 15, 2014. http://www.newyorker.com/magazine/2014/09/15/transformation-3.

ADDITIONAL SOURCES

"About blood and marrow transplantation." Memorial Sloan Kettering Cancer Center. Accessed March 9, 2017. https://www.mskcc.org/pediatrics/cancer-care/treatments/cancer-treatments/transplantation/about.

Ballen, Karen K. "Is There a Best Graft Source of Transplantation in Acute Myeloid Leukemia?" *Best Practice & Research Clinical Haematology* 28, no. 2-3 (2015): 147–54. https://doi.org/10.1016/j.beha.2015.10.012.

"Bone marrow transplantation." MedlinePlus. January 12, 2017. https://medlineplus.gov/bonemarrowtransplantation.html.

Dykewicz, Clare A. "Hospital Infection Control in Hematopoietic Stem Cell Transplant Recipients." *Emerging Infectious Diseases,* 7, no 2 (2001): 263–67. https://doi.org/10.3201/eid0702.700263.

Dykewicz, Clare A. "Summary of the Guidelines for Preventing Opportunistic Infections among Hematopoietic Stem Cell Transplant Recipients." *Clinical Infectious Diseases* 33, no. 2 (2001): 139–44. https://doi.org/10.1086/321805.

Gaballa, Sameh, Neil Palmisiano, Onder Alpdogan, Matthew Carabasi, Joanne Filicko-O'Hara, Margaret Kasner, Walter K. Kraft, Benjamin Leiby, Ubaldo Martinez-Outschoorn, William O'Hara, et al. "A Two-Step Haploidentical versus a Two-Step Matched Related Allogeneic Myeloablative Peripheral Blood Stem Cell Transplantation." *Biology of Blood and Marrow Transplantation: Journal of the American Society for Blood and Marrow Transplantation,* 22, no. 1 (2016): 141–48. https://doi.org/10.1016/j.bbmt.2015.09.017.

"Graft-versus-host disease." Be the Match. November 30, 2016. https://bethematch.org/for-patients-and-families/life-after-transplant/graft-versus-host-disease--gvhd-/.

Grosso, Dolores, Sameh Gaballa, Onder Alpdogan, Matthew Carabasi, Joanne Filicko-O'Hara, Margaret Kasner, Ubaldo Martinez-Outschoorn, John L. Wagner, William O'Hara, Shannon Rudolph, et al. "A Two-Step Approach to Myeloablative Haploidentical Transplantation: Low Nonrelapse Mortality and High Survival Confirmed in Patients with Earlier Stage Disease." *Biology of Blood and Marrow Transplantation* 21, no. 4 (2015): 646–52. https://doi.org/10.1016/j.bbmt.2014.12.019.

"Hand hygiene in healthcare settings." Centers for Disease Control and Prevention. Accessed March 9, 2017. https://www.cdc.gov/handhygiene/.

"Handwashing videos—CDC." Centers for Disease Control and Prevention. Accessed March 9, 2017. https://www.cdc.gov/handwashing/videos.html.

"Handwashing: Clean hands save lives." Centers for Disease Control and Prevention. February 15, 2017. https://www.cdc.gov/handwashing/when-how-handwashing.html.

REFERENCES

"Infection prevention." Be the Match. December 23, 2014. https://bethematch.org/for-patients-and-families/life-after-transplant/staying-healthy/infection-prevention/

Isoyama, K., M. Oda, K. Kato, T. Nagamura-Inoue, S. Kai, H. Kigasawa, R. Kobayashi, J. Mimaya, M. Inoue, A. Kikuchi, et al. "Long-Term Outcome of Cord Blood Transplantation from Unrelated Donors as an Initial Transplantation Procedure for Children with AML in Japan." *Bone Marrow Transplantation* 45, no. 1 (2009): 69–77. https://doi.org/10.1038/bmt.2009.93.

Rich, Ivan N. "Improving Quality and Potency Testing for Umbilical Cord Blood: A New Perspective." *STEM CELLS Translational Medicine* 4, no. 9 (2015): 967–73. https://doi.org/10.5966/sctm.2015-0036.

Rosenberg, N.and R. R. Nelson. "American Universities and Technical Advance in Industry." *Research Policy*, 23, no. 3 (1994): 323–48.

"StatBite AML Survival after Bone Marrow Transplant by Type of Donor." *JNCI Journal of the National Cancer Institute* 103, no. 10 (2011): 783–83. https://doi.org/10.1093/jnci/djr179.

"Transplant Frequently Asked Questions." US Department of Health and Human Services. Accessed March 9, 2017. https://bloodcell.transplant.hrsa.gov/transplant/understanding_tx/transplant_faqs/index.html.

"WHO Guidelines on Hand Hygiene in Health Care: First Global Patient Safety Challenge: Clean Care Is Safer Care." World Health Organization. 2010.

Young, Jo-Anne H., Brent R. Logan, Juan Wu, John R. Wingard, Daniel J. Weisdorf, Cathryn Mudrick, Kristin Knust, Mary M. Horowitz, Dennis L. Confer, Erik R. Dubberke, et al. "Infections after Transplantation of Bone Marrow or Peripheral Blood Stem Cells from Unrelated Donors." *Biology of Blood and Marrow Transplantation* 22, no. 2 (2016): 359–70. https://doi.org/10.1016/j.bbmt.2015.09.013.

SEEKING CONTROL

A lawsuit that they won against Genentech:

Pollack, Andrew. "A Jury Orders Genentech to Pay $300 Million in Royalties," *New York Times,* June 11, 2002. https://www.nytimes.com/2002/06/11/business/a-jury-orders-genentech-to-pay-300-million-in-royalties.html.

Receive related transplants:

Hede, K. "Half-Match Bone Marrow Transplants May Raise Odds for More Recipients." *JNCI Journal of the National Cancer Institute* 103, no. 10 (2011): 781–83. https://doi.org/10.1093/jnci/djr181.

Large volumes of healthy stem cells:

Ballen, Karen K. "Is There a Best Graft Source of Transplantation in Acute Myeloid Leukemia?" *Best Practice & Research Clinical Haematology* 28, no. 2-3 (2015): 147–54. https://doi.org/10.1016/j.beha.2015.10.012.

See also: Gaballa, Sameh, Neil Palmisiano, Onder Alpdogan, Matthew Carabasi, Joanne Filicko-O'Hara, Margaret Kasner, Walter K. Kraft, Benjamin Leiby, Ubaldo Martinez-Outschoorn, William O'Hara et al. "A Two-Step Haploidentical versus a Two-Step Matched Related Allogeneic Myeloablative Peripheral Blood Stem Cell Transplantation." *Biology of Blood and Marrow Transplantation: Journal of the American Society for Blood and Marrow Transplantation,* 22, no1 (2016): 141–48. https://doi.org/10.1016/j.bbmt.2015.09.017

The absence of matched donors:

Isoyama, K., M. Oda, K. Kato, T. Nagamura-Inoue, S. Kai, H. Kigasawa, R. Kobayashi, J. Mimaya, M. Inoue, A. Kikuchi, et al. "Long-Term Outcome of Cord Blood Transplantation from Unrelated Donors as an Initial Transplantation Procedure for Children with AML in Japan." *Bone Marrow Transplantation* 45, no. 1 (2009): 69–77. https://doi.org/10.1038/bmt.2009.93.

See also: Munoz, Javier, Nina Shah, Katayoun Rezvani, Chitra Hosing, Catherine M. Bollard, Betul Oran, Amanda Olson, Uday Popat, Jeffrey Molldrem, Ian K. Mcniece et al. "Concise Review: Umbilical Cord Blood Transplantation: Past, Present, and Future." *STEM CELLS Translational Medicine* 3, no. 12 (2014): 1435–43.

Sanz, Jaime, Miguel A. Sanz, Silvana Saavedra, Ignacio Lorenzo, Pau Montesinos, Leonor Senent, Dolores Planelles, Luis Larrea, Guillermo Martín, Javier Palau et al. "Cord Blood Transplantation from Unrelated Donors in Adults with High-Risk Acute Myeloid Leukemia." *Biology of Blood and Marrow Transplantation* 16, no. 1 (2010): 86–94.

Sato, A., J. Ooi, S. Takahashi, N. Tsukada, S. Kato, T. Kawakita, T. Yagyu, F. Nagamura, T. Iseki, A. Tojo, et al. "Unrelated Cord Blood Transplantation after Myeloablative Conditioning in Adults with Advanced Myelodysplastic Syndromes." *Bone Marrow Transplantation* 46, no. 2 (2010): 257–61.

ADDITIONAL SOURCES

"City of Hope v. Genentech." April 24, 2008. Stanford Law School, Robert Crown Library. http://scocal.stanford.edu/opinion/city-hope-v-genentech-33188.

Ciurea, Stefan O., Mei-Jie Zhang, Andrea A. Bacigalupo, Asad Bashey, Frederick R. Appelbaum, Omar S. Aljitawi, Philippe Armand, Joseph H. Antin, Junfang Chen, Steven M. Devine, et al. "Haploidentical Transplant with Posttransplant Cyclophosphamide vs. Matched Unrelated Donor Transplant for Acute Myeloid Leukemia." *Blood* 126, no. 8 (2015): 1033–40. https://doi.org/10.1182/blood-2015-04-639831.

"Genentech reports 28 percent increase in product sales for second quarter." Genentech. July 10, 2002. https://www.gene.com/media/press-releases/5227/2002-07-10/genentech-reports-28-percent-increase-in.

Haw, Jennie. "From Waste to (Fool's) Gold: Promissory and Profit Values of Cord Blood." *Monash Bioethics Review* 33, no. 4 (2015): 325–39. https://doi.org/10.1007/s40592-015-0048-5.

Hede, K. "Half-Match Bone Marrow Transplants May Raise Odds for More Recipients." *JNCI Journal of the National Cancer Institute* 103, no. 10 (2011): 781–83. https://doi.org/10.1093/jnci/djr181.

Matsumoto, Monica M. and Kirstin R. W. Matthews. "A Need for Renewed and Cohesive US Policy on Cord Blood Banking." *Stem Cell Reviews and Reports* 11, no. 6 (2015): 789–97. https://doi.org/10.1007/s12015-015-9613-9.

Munoz, Javier, Nina Shah, Katayoun Rezvani, Chitra Hosing, Catherine M. Bollard, Betul Oran, Amanda Olson, Uday Popat, Jeffrey Molldrem, Ian K. Mcniece et al. "Concise Review: Umbilical Cord Blood Transplantation: Past, Present, and Future." *STEM CELLS Translational Medicine* 3, no. 12 (2014): 1435–43. https://doi.org/10.5966/sctm.2014-0151.

Pollack, Andrew. "A Jury Orders Genentech to Pay $300 Million in Royalties," *New York Times*, June 11, 2002. https://www.nytimes.com/2002/06/11/business/a-jury-orders-genentech-to-pay-300-million-in-royalties.html.

Sanz, Jaime, Miguel A. Sanz, Silvana Saavedra, Ignacio Lorenzo, Pau Montesinos, Leonor Senent, Dolores Planelles, Luis Larrea, Guillermo Martín, Javier Palau et al. "Cord Blood Transplantation from Unrelated Donors in Adults with High-Risk Acute Myeloid Leukemia." *Biology of Blood and Marrow Transplantation* 16, no. 1 (2010): 86–94. https://doi.org/10.1016/j.bbmt.2009.09.001.

Sato, A, J Ooi, S. Takahashi, N. Tsukada, S. Kato, T. Kawakita, T. Yagyu, F. Nagamura, T. Iseki, A. Tojo, et al. "Unrelated Cord Blood Transplantation after Myeloablative Conditioning in Adults with Advanced Myelodysplastic Syndromes." *Bone Marrow Transplantation* 46, no. 2 (2010): 257–61. https://doi.org/10.1038/bmt.2010.91.

CHAPTER FIVE: TRANSPLANT/SECOND VISIT

This avoidance applies both to patients and their doctors:

Baszanger, Isabelle. "One More Chemo or One Too Many? Defining the Limits of Treatment and Innovation in Medical Oncology." *Social Science & Medicine* 75, no. 5 (2012): 864–72.

See also: Fattoum, Jihane, Giovanna Cannas, Mohamed Elhamri, Isabelle Tigaud, Adriana Plesa, Maël Heiblig, Claudiu Plesa, Eric Wattel, and Xavier Thomas. "Effect of Age on Treatment Decision-Making in Elderly Patients with Acute Myeloid Leukemia." *Clinical Lymphoma Myeloma and Leukemia* 15, no. 8 (2015): 477–83.

Leblanc, Thomas W., Laura J. Fish, Catherine T. Bloom, Areej El-Jawahri, Debra M. Davis, Susan C. Locke, Karen E. Steinhauser, and Kathryn I. Pollak. "Patient Experiences of Acute Myeloid Leukemia: A Qualitative Study about Diagnosis, Illness Understanding, and Treatment Decision-Making." *Psycho-Oncology* 26, no. 12 (2016): 2063–68.

Magarotto, Roberto, Gianluigi Lunardi, Francesca Coati, Paola Cassandrini, Vincenzo Picece, Silvia Ferrighi, Luciana Oliosi, and Marco Venturini. "Reduced Use of Chemotherapy at the End of Life in an Integrated-Care Model of Oncology and Palliative Care. *Tumori*, 97, no. 5 (2011): 573–77.

ADDITIONAL SOURCES

Baccarani, M., F. Efficace, and G. Rosti. "Moving towards Patient-Centered Decision-Making in Chronic Myeloid Leukemia: Assessment of Quality of Life and Symptom Burden." *Haematologica* 99, no. 2 (2014): 205–08. https://doi.org/10.3324/haematol.2013.094045.

Baszanger, Isabelle. "One More Chemo or One Too Many? Defining the Limits of Treatment and Innovation in Medical Oncology." *Social Science & Medicine* 75, no. 5 (2012): 864–72. https://doi.org/10.1016/j.socscimed.2012.03.023.

Chambaere, Kenneth, Johan Bilsen, Joachim Cohen, Geert Pousset, Bregje Onwuteaka-Philipsen, Freddy Mortier, and Luc Deliens. "A Post-Mortem Survey on End-of-Life Decisions Using a Representative Sample of Death Certificates in Flanders, Belgium: Research Protocol." *BMC Public Health* 8, no. 1 (2008). https://doi.org/10.1186/1471-2458-8-299.

Chambaere, Kenneth, Judith Ac Rietjens, Joachim Cohen, Koen Pardon, Reginald Deschepper, H. Roeline, W. Pasman, and Luc Deliens. "Is Educational Attainment Related to End-of-Life Decision-Making? A Large Post-Mortem Survey in Belgium." *BMC Public Health* 13, no. 1 (2013). https://doi.org/10.1186/1471-2458-13-1055.

Deschler, B., T. de Witte, R. Mertelsmann, and M. Lübbert. "Treatment Decision-Making for Older Patients with High-Risk Myelodysplastic Syndrome or Acute Myeloid Leukemia: Problems and Approaches." *Haematologica*, 91, no. 11 (2006): 1513–22.

Efficace, Fabio, Georg Kemmler, Marco Vignetti, Franco Mandelli, Stefano Molica, and Bernhard Holzner. "Health-Related Quality of Life Assessment and Reported Outcomes in Leukaemia Randomised Controlled Trials—A Systematic Review to Evaluate the Added Value in Supporting Clinical Decision Making." *European Journal of Cancer* 44, no. 11 (2008): 1497–1506. https://doi.org/10.1016/j.ejca.2008.03.017.

Fattoum, Jihane, Giovanna Cannas, Mohamed Elhamri, Isabelle Tigaud, Adriana Plesa, Maël Heiblig, Claudiu Plesa, Eric Wattel, and Xavier Thomas. "Effect of Age on Treatment Decision-Making in Elderly Patients with Acute Myeloid Leukemia." *Clinical Lymphoma Myeloma and Leukemia* 15, no. 8 (2015): 477–83. https://doi.org/10.1016/j.clml.2015.02.022.

Fins, Joseph J. and Mildred Z. Solomon. "Communication in Intensive Care Settings: The Challenge of Futility Disputes." *Critical Care Medicine* 29, no. Supplement (2001). https://doi.org/10.1097/00003246-200102001-00003.

Jones, James W. and Laurence B. Mccullough. "Extending Life or Prolonging Death: When Is Enough Actually Too Much?" *Journal of Vascular Surgery* 60, no. 2 (2014): 521–22. https://doi.org/10.1016/j.jvs.2014.05.054.

Jukić, Marko. "Medical Futility Treatment in Intensive Care Units." *Acta Medica Academica* 45, no. 2 (2016): 127–36. https://doi.org/10.5644/ama2006-124.169.

Lancet, The. "Balancing the Benefits and Risks of Choice." *The Lancet* 388, no. 10050 (2016): 1129. https://doi.org/10.1016/s0140-6736(16)31641-5.

Leblanc, Thomas W., Laura J. Fish, Catherine T. Bloom, Areej El-Jawahri, Debra M. Davis, Susan C. Locke, Karen E. Steinhauser, and Kathryn I. Pollak. "Patient Experiences of Acute Myeloid Leukemia: A Qualitative Study about Diagnosis, Illness Understanding, and Treatment Decision-Making." *Psycho-Oncology* 26, no. 12 (2016): 2063–68. https://doi.org/10.1002/pon.4309.

Magarotto, Roberto, Gianluigi Lunardi, Francesca Coati, Paola Cassandrini, Vincenzo Picece, Silvia Ferrighi, Luciana Oliosi, and Marco Venturini. "Reduced Use of Chemotherapy at the End of Life in an Integrated-Care Model of Oncology and Palliative Care. *Tumori*, 97, no. 5 (2011): 573–77. https://doi.org/10.1700/989.10714.

Miller, Kimberly D., Rebecca L. Siegel, Chun Chieh Lin, Angela B. Mariotto, Joan L. Kramer, Julia H. Rowland, Kevin D. Stein, Rick Alteri, and Ahmedin Jemal. "Cancer Treatment and Survivorship Statistics, 2016." *CA: A Cancer Journal for Clinicians* 66, no. 4 (2016): 271–89. https://doi.org/10.3322/caac.21349.

Myers, G. "Over-Medicalized Care at the End-of-Life in the United States." Turn-Key Health. December 2016. http://turn-keyhealth.com/wp-content/uploads/2016/12/Over-Medicalized-Care-at-the-End-of-Life-in-the-US.pdf.

Pardon, Koen, Kenneth Chambaere, H. Roeline W. Pasman, Reginald Deschepper, Judith Rietjens, and Luc Deliens. "Trends in End-of-Life Decision Making in Patients with and without Cancer." *Journal of Clinical Oncology* 31, no. 11 (2013): 1450–57. https://doi.org/10.1200/jco.2012.44.5916.

Rood, Janneke A. J., Florence J. Van Zuuren, Frank Stam, Tjeerd Van Der Ploeg, Corien Eeltink, Irma M. Verdonck-De Leeuw, and Peter C. Huijgens. "Perceived Need for Information among Patients with a Haematological Malignancy: Associations with Information Satisfaction and Treatment Decision-Making Preferences." *Hematological Oncology* 33, no. 2 (2014): 85–98. https://doi.org/10.1002/hon.2138.

Smith, Martin L. "Should Possible Disparities and Distrust Trump Do-No-Harm?" *The American Journal of Bioethics* 6, no. 5 (2006): 28–30. https://doi.org/10.1080/15265160600860860.

Solomon, M. Z., L. O'donnell, B. Jennings, V. Guilfoy, S. M. Wolf, K. Nolan, R. Jackson, D. Koch-Weser, and S. Donnelley. "Decisions near the End of Life: Professional Views on Life-Sustaining Treatments." *American Journal of Public Health* 83, no. 1 (1993): 14–23. https://doi.org/10.2105/ajph.83.1.14.

Waldrop, D. P., and M. A. Meeker. "Hospice Decision Making: Diagnosis Makes a Difference." *The Gerontologist* 52, no. 5 (2012): 686–97. https://doi.org/10.1093/geront/gnr160.

Wojtasiewicz, Mary Ellen. "Damage Compounded: Disparities, Distrust, and Disparate Impact in End-of-Life Conflict Resolution Policies." *The American Journal of Bioethics* 6, no. 5 (2006): 8–12. https://doi.org/10.1080/15265160600856801.

CHAPTER SIX: LEUKEMIA RETURNS

"Acute myeloid leukemia (AML)." DynaMed. 2016. http://search.ebscohost.com/login.aspx?direct=true&db=dnh&AN=114798&site=dynamed-live&scope=site. Registration and login required.

"Acute Myeloid Leukemia—Cancer Stat Facts." National Cancer Institute. 2012. https://seer.cancer.gov/statfacts/html/amyl.html.

Alatrash, Gheath, Matteo Pelosini, Rima M. Saliba, Ebru Koca, Gabriela Rondon, Borje S. Andersson, Alexandre Chiattone, Weiqing Zhang, Sergio A. Giralt, and Amanda M. Cernosek. "Platelet Recovery Before Allogeneic Stem Cell Transplantation Predicts Posttransplantation Outcomes in Patients with Acute Myelogenous Leukemia and Myelodysplastic Syndrome." *Biology of Blood and Marrow Transplantation* 17, no. 12 (2011): 1841–45. https://doi.org/10.1016/j.bbmt.2011.05.018.

Chang, Hui-Yen, Victorio Rodriguez, Gino Narboni, Gerald P. Bodey, Mario A. Luna, and Emil J. Freireich. "Causes of Death in Adults with Acute Leukemia." *Medicine* 55, no. 3 (1976): 259–68. https://doi.org/10.1097/00005792-197605000-00005.

Ferrara, Felicetto and Charles A Schiffer. "Acute Myeloid Leukaemia in Adults." *The Lancet* 381, no. 9865 (2013): 484–95. https://doi.org/10.1016/s0140-6736(12)61727-9.

Fey, M.F and C. Buske. "Acute Myeloblastic Leukaemias in Adult Patients: ESMO Clinical Practice Guidelines for Diagnosis, Treatment and Follow-Up." *Annals of Oncology* 24 (2013): vii138–vii143. https://doi.org/10.1093/annonc/mdt320.

Huck, Amelia, Olga Pozdnyakova, Andrew Brunner, John M. Higgins, Amir T. Fathi, and Robert P. Hasserjian. "Prior Cytopenia Predicts Worse Clinical Outcome in Acute Myeloid Leukemia." *Leukemia Research* 39, no. 10 (2015): 1034–40. https://doi.org/10.1016/j.leukres.2015.06.012.

Lai, Xin and Kelvin K. W. Yau. "Long-Term Survivor Model with Bivariate Random Effects: Applications to Bone Marrow Transplant and Carcinoma Study Data." *Statistics in Medicine* 27, no. 27 (2008): 5692–08. https://doi.org/10.1002/sim.3404.

Milligan, D. W., D. Grimwade, J. O. Cullis, L. Bond, D. Swirsky, C. Craddock, J. Kell, J. Homewood, K. Campbell, and S. Mcginley. "Guidelines on the Management of Acute Myeloid Leukaemia in Adults." *British Journal of Haematology* 135, no. 4 (2006): 450–74. https://doi.org/10.1111/j.1365-2141.2006.06314.x.

O'Donnell, M. R., M. S Tallman, C. N. Abboud, J. Altman, F.R. Appelbaum, V. Bhatt, et al. "NCCN guidelines version 1.2017 acute myeloid leukemia." February 2007. https://www.nccn.org/professionals/physician_gls/f_guidelines.asp.

Saliba, R. M., K. V. Komanduri, S. Giralt, J. De Souza, P. Patah, B. Oran, D. Couriel, G. Rondon, R. E. Champlin, and M. De Lima. "Leukemia Burden Delays Lymphocyte and Platelet Recovery after Allo-SCT for AML." *Bone Marrow Transplantation* 43, no. 9 (2008): 685–92. https://doi.org/10.1038/bmt.2008.376.

Siegel, Bernie S. *A Book of Miracles: Inspiring True Stories of Healing, Gratitude, and Love.* Novato, California: New World Library, 2011.

Siegel, Bernie S. *Love, Medicine and Miracles.* London: Arrow, 1988.

Tallman, Martin S., Waleska S. Pérez, Hillard M. Lazarus, Robert Peter Gale, Richard T. Maziarz, Jacob M. Rowe, David I. Marks, Jean-Yves Cahn, Asad Bashey, and Michael R. Bishop. "Pretransplantation Consolidation Chemotherapy Decreases Leukemia Relapse after Autologous Blood and Bone Marrow Transplants for Acute Myelogenous Leukemia in First Remission." *Biology of Blood and Marrow Transplantation* 12, no. 2 (2006): 204–16. https://doi.org/10.1016/j.bbmt.2005.10.013.

Trafalis, Dimitrios, Elias Poulakidas, Violeta Kapsimali, Christos Tsigris, Xenofon Papanicolaou, Nikolaos Harhalakis, Emmanuel Nikiforakis, and Chrisanthi Mentzikof-Mitsouli. "Platelet Production and Related Pathophysiology in Acute Myelogenous Leukemia at First Diagnosis: Prognostic Implications." *Oncology Reports*, 2008. https://doi.org/10.3892/or.19.4.1021.

IN MEMORIAM

Four percent three-year survival after early relapse:

Bejanyan, Nelli, Daniel J. Weisdorf, Brent R. Logan, Hai-Lin Wang, Steven M. Devine, Marcos De Lima, Donald W. Bunjes, and Mei-Jie Zhang. "Survival of Patients with Acute Myeloid Leukemia Relapsing after Allogeneic Hematopoietic Cell Transplantation: A Center for International Blood and Marrow Transplant Research Study." *Biology of Blood and Marrow Transplantation* 21, no. 3 (2015): 454–59. https://doi.org/10.1016/j.bbmt.2014.11.007.

One of the great cancer success stories:

Hunger, Stephen P., Xiaomin Lu, Meenakshi Devidas, Bruce M. Camitta, Paul S. Gaynon, Naomi J. Winick, Gregory H. Reaman, and William L. Carroll. "Improved Survival for Children and Adolescents with Acute Lymphoblastic Leukemia Between 1990 and 2005: A Report from the Children's Oncology Group." *Journal of Clinical Oncology* 30, no. 14 (2012): 1663–69. https://doi.org/10.1200/jco.2011.37.8018.

ADDITIONAL SOURCES

"Cancer immunotherapy." MedlinePlus. Accessed March 21, 2017. https://medlineplus.gov/cancerimmunotherapy.html.

Chang, Wen-Pei and Chia-Chin Lin. "Correlation between Rest-Activity Rhythm and Survival in Cancer Patients Experiencing Pain." *Chronobiology International* 31, no. 8 (2014): 926–34. https://doi.org/10.3109/07420528.2014.931412.

Devlin, Ann Sloan, and Allison B. Arneill. "Health Care Environments and Patient Outcomes." *Environment and Behavior* 35, no. 5 (2003): 665–94. https://doi.org/10.1177/0013916503255102.

"Facts 2014–2015." Leukemia and Lymphoma Society. 2015. https://www.lls.org/sites/default/files/file_assets/facts.pdf.

"Fatigue." National Cancer Institute. January 13, 2017. https://www.cancer.gov/about-cancer/treatment/side-effects/fatigue/fatigue-hp-pdq.

Fouladiun, M., U. Korner, L. Gunnebo, P. Sixt-Ammilon, I. Bosaeus, and K. Lundholm. "Daily Physical-Rest Activities in Relation to Nutritional State, Metabolism, and Quality of Life in Cancer Patients with Progressive Cachexia." *Clinical Cancer Research* 13, no. 21 (2007): 6379–85. https://doi.org/10.1158/1078-0432.ccr-07-1147.

Huisman, E.R.C.M., E. Morales, J. Van Hoof, and H.S.M. Kort. "Healing Environment: A Review of the Impact of Physical Environmental Factors on Users." *Building and Environment* 58 (2012): 70–80. https://doi.org/10.1016/j.buildenv.2012.06.016.

Hunger, Stephen P., Xiaomin Lu, Meenakshi Devidas, Bruce M. Camitta, Paul S. Gaynon, Naomi J. Winick, Gregory H. Reaman, and William L. Carroll. "Improved Survival for Children and Adolescents with Acute Lymphoblastic Leukemia Between 1990 and 2005: A Report from the Children's Oncology Group." *Journal of Clinical Oncology* 30, no. 14 (2012): 1663–69. https://doi.org/10.1200/jco.2011.37.8018.

"Immunotherapy." National Cancer Institute. Accessed March 21, 2017. https://www.cancer.gov/about-cancer/treatment/types/immunotherapy.

Miaskowski, Christine, Kathryn Lee, Laura Dunn, Marylin Dodd, Bradley E. Aouizerat, Claudia West, Steven M. Paul, Bruce Cooper, William Wara, and Patrick Swift. "Sleep-Wake Circadian Activity Rhythm Parameters and Fatigue in Oncology Patients Before the Initiation of Radiation Therapy." *Cancer Nursing* 34, no. 4 (2011): 255–68. https://doi.org/10.1097/ncc.0b013e3181f65d9b.

Snook, A. E. and S. A. Waldman. Advances in cancer immunotherapy. *Discovery*, 15, no. 81 (2013): 120–25.

part three

CHAPTER EIGHT: DOCTORS SPEAK

Disengagement, substance abuse, early retirement, or burnout:

Drummond, Dike. *Stop Physician Burnout: What to Do When Working Harder Isn't Working.* Heritage Press Publications, 2014.

See also Peckham, C. "Medscape Lifestyle Report 2017: Race and Ethnicity, Bias and Burnout" (2017) 1–28. Accessed at http://www.medscape.com/features/slideshow/lifestyle/2017/overview.

CHAPTER NINE: PATIENTS SPEAK

Decrease blood pressure and induce relaxation in patients:

Mitrione, Stephen. (2008). "Therapeutic Responses to Natural Environments: Using Gardens to Improve Health Care." *Minnesota Medicine*, 91, no. 3(2008): 31–34.

A view of a brick wall:

Ulrich, Roger S. (2002). "Health Benefits of Gardens in Hospitals." Citeseer. In paper for conference. Plants for People International Exhibition Floriade, 17, p. 2010. Citeseer. http://citeseerx.ist.psu.edu/viewdoc/download?doi=10.1.1.541.4830&rep=rep1&type=pdf.

Derive substantial benefit:

Franklin, D. (2012). "Nature that nurtures." *Scientific American*, 306, no. 3 (2012): 24–25.

For our mental and physical health:

Reynolds, G. "How walking in nature changes the brain," *New York Times*, July 22, 2015. https://well.blogs.nytimes.com/2015/07/22/how-nature-changes-the-brain/.

Exposure to nature decreases depression:

Schweitzer, Marc, Laura Gilpin, and Susan Frampton. "Healing Spaces: Elements of Environmental Design That Make an Impact on Health." *The Journal of Alternative and Complementary Medicine* 10, no. 1 (2004): 71–83.

See also Tamjidi, Z., A. Hajian, and B. Ghafourian. (2016). "Healing Garden: Study of the Therapeutic Effects of the Natural Environment in Pediatric Hospital." *Journal of Current Research in Science; Tabriz*, 4, no. 3 (2016): 152–59.

REFERENCES

Exposure to urban environments:

Bratman, Gregory N., J. Paul Hamilton, Kevin S. Hahn, Gretchen C. Daily, and James J. Gross. "Nature Experience Reduces Rumination and Subgenual Prefrontal Cortex Activation." *Proceedings of the National Academy of Sciences* 112, no. 28 (2015): 8567–72. https://doi.org/10.1073/pnas.1510459112.

ADDITIONAL SOURCES

"Aidan in Prouty Garden at Children's Hospital Boston," filmed August 22, 2011. heartofboston268, video, 10:03, https://www.youtube.com/watch?v=gea7au2CL9Y.

Aoki, Jun, Heiwa Kanamori, Masatsugu Tanaka, Satoshi Yamasaki, Takahiro Fukuda, Hiroyasu Ogawa, Koji Iwato, Kazuteru Ohashi, Hirokazu Okumura, Makoto Onizuka et al. "Impact of Age on Outcomes of Allogeneic Hematopoietic Stem Cell Transplantation with Reduced Intensity Conditioning in Elderly Patients with Acute Myeloid Leukemia." *American Journal of Hematology* 91, no. 3 (2016): 302–7. https://doi.org/10.1002/ajh.24270.

Bejanyan, Nelli, Daniel J. Weisdorf, Brent R. Logan, Hai-Lin Wang, Steven M. Devine, Marcos De Lima, Donald W. Bunjes, and Mei-Jie Zhang. "Survival of Patients with Acute Myeloid Leukemia Relapsing after Allogeneic Hematopoietic Cell Transplantation: A Center for International Blood and Marrow Transplant Research Study." *Biology of Blood and Marrow Transplantation* 21, no. 3 (2015): 454–59. https://doi.org/10.1016/j.bbmt.2014.11.007.

Bratman, Gregory N., J. Paul Hamilton, Kevin S. Hahn, Gretchen C. Daily, and James J. Gross. "Nature Experience Reduces Rumination and Subgenual Prefrontal Cortex Activation." *Proceedings of the National Academy of Sciences* 112, no. 28 (2015): 8567–72. https://doi.org/10.1073/pnas.1510459112.

Broglie, Larisa, Irene Helenowski, Lawrence J. Jennings, Kristian Schafernak, Reggie Duerst, Jennifer Schneiderman, William Tse, Morris Kletzel, and Sonali Chaudhury. "Early Mixed T-Cell Chimerism Is Predictive of Pediatric AML or MDS Relapse after Hematopoietic Stem Cell Transplant." *Pediatric Blood & Cancer* 64, no. 9 (2017). https://doi.org/10.1002/pbc.26493.

Carmel-Gilfilen, Candy and Margaret Portillo. "Designing with Empathy." *HERD: Health Environments Research & Design Journal* 9, no. 2 (2015): 130–46. https://doi.org/10.1177/1937586715592633.

Franklin, D. "Nature That Nurtures." *Scientific American*, 306, no. 3 (2012): 24–25.

Hartig, Terry and Clare Cooper Marcus. "Essay: Healing Gardens—Places for Nature in Health Care." *The Lancet* 368 (2006). https://doi.org/10.1016/s0140-6736(06)69920-0.

Lim, Sara J., Matthew J. Lim, Anastasios Raptis, Jing-Zhou Hou, Rafic Farah, Stanley M. Marks, Annie Im, Kathleen Dorritie, Alison Sehgal, Mounzer Agha et al. "Inferior Outcome after Allogeneic Transplant in First Remission in High-Risk AML Patients Who Required More than Two Cycles of Induction Therapy." *American Journal of Hematology* 90, no. 8 (2015): 715–18. https://doi.org/10.1002/ajh.24062.

Marcus, Clare Cooper and Marnie Barnes. "Gardens in Healthcare Facilities: Uses, Therapeutic Benefits, and Design Recommendations." Martinez, CA: Center for Health Design, 1995.

Marcus, Clare Cooper. "The Future of Healing Gardens." *HERD: Health Environments Research & Design Journal* 9, no. 2 (2015): 172–74. https://doi.org/10.1177/1937586715606926.

Mccaffrey, Ruth. "The Effect of Healing Gardens and Art Therapy on Older Adults with Mild to Moderate Depression." *Holistic Nursing Practice* 21, no. 2 (2007): 79–84. https://doi.org/10.1097/01.hnp.0000262022.80044.06.

Milligan, Christine, Anthony Gatrell, and Amanda Bingley. "'Cultivating Health': Therapeutic Landscapes and Older People in Northern England." *Social Science & Medicine* 58, no. 9 (2004): 1781–93. https://doi.org/10.1016/s0277-9536(03)00397-6.

Mitrione, Stephen. "Therapeutic Responses to Natural Environments: Using Gardens to Improve Health Care." *Minnesota Medicine*, 91, no. 3 (2008): 31–34.

Park, Sang Hyuk, Chan-Jeoung Park, Borae G. Park, Mi-Hyun Bae, Bo-Hyun Kim, Young-Uk Cho, Seongsoo Jang, Ae-Ja Park, Dae-Young Kim, and Jung-Hee Lee. "Prognostic Impact of Lymphocyte Subpopulations in Peripheral Blood after Hematopoietic Stem Cell Transplantation for Hematologic Malignancies." *Cytometry Part B: Clinical Cytometry* 94, no. 2 (2017): 270–80. https://doi.org/10.1002/cyto.b.21510.

Rashidi, Armin, Maryam Ebadi, Graham A. Colditz, and John F. Dipersio. "Outcomes of Allogeneic Stem Cell Transplantation in Elderly Patients with Acute Myeloid Leukemia: A Systematic Review and Meta-Analysis." *Biology of Blood and Marrow Transplantation* 22, no. 4 (2016): 651–57. https://doi.org/10.1016/j.bbmt.2015.10.019.

Reynolds, G. "How walking in nature changes the brain." Retrieved May 4, 2017, from https://well.blogs.nytimes.com/2015/07/22/how-nature-changes-the-brain/.

Rodiek, S. and C. Lee. Elderly care: Increasing outdoor usage in residential facilities. *World Health Design, Gateways to Health,* (2009): 49–55.

Schweitzer, Marc, Laura Gilpin, and Susan Frampton. "Healing Spaces: Elements of Environmental Design That Make an Impact on Health." *The Journal of Alternative and Complementary Medicine* 10, no. 1 (2004): 71–83. https://doi.org/10.1089/1075553042245953.

Sherman, Sandra A., James W. Varni, Roger S. Ulrich, and Vanessa L. Malcarne. "Post-Occupancy Evaluation of Healing Gardens in a Pediatric Cancer Center." *Landscape and Urban Planning* 73, no. 2-3 (2005): 167–83. https://doi.org/10.1016/j.landurbplan.2004.11.013.

Sternberg, E. M. *Healing Spaces: The Science of Place and Well-Being*. Cambridge, MA: Belknap Press, 2010.

Tamjidi, Z., A. Hajian, and B. Ghafourian. "Healing Garden: Study of the Therapeutic Effects of the Natural Environment in Pediatric Hospital." *Journal of Current Research in Science; Tabriz*, 4, no. 3 (2016): 152–59.

Ulrich, Roger S. "View through a Window May Influence Recovery from Surgery." *Science*, 224, 4647 (1984): 420–21.

Ulrich, Roger S. (2002). "Health Benefits of Gardens in Hospitals." Citeseer. In paper for conference. Plants for People International Exhibition Floriade, 17, p. 2010. http://citeseerx.ist.psu.edu/viewdoc/download?doi=10.1.1.541.4830&rep=rep1&type=pdf.

"Work increasing for landscape architecture firms, survey shows." American Society of Landscape Architects, July 28, 2011. https://www.asla.org/NewsReleaseDetails.aspx?id=32424

part four

CHAPTER TEN: FROM EMOTIONAL ARMOR TO EMOTIONAL AGILITY

David, Susan. *Emotional Agility: Get Unstuck, Embrace Change, and Thrive in Work and Life*. New York: Avery, 2016.

Riess, Helen. *The Empathy Effect: Seven Neuroscience-Based Keys for Transforming the Way We Live, Love, Work, and Connect Across Differences*. Louisville, CO: Sounds True, 2018.

CHAPTER ELEVEN: ENHANCING PALLIATIVE CARE

Our culture has systematically removed death from everyday life:

Johnson, J. "Why We Need to Talk about Death and Dying," *Huffington Post*, August 17, 2010. http://www.huffingtonpost.com/judith-johnson/why-we-need-to-talk-about_b_682218.html.

See also Khullar, Dhruv. "We're bad at death. Can we talk?" *New York Times*, May 10, 2017. https://www.nytimes.com/2017/05/10/upshot/were-bad-at-death-first-we-need-a-good-talk.html.

The same desire to die at home as do patients with greater social support:

Aoun, Samar M., Lauren J. Breen, and Denise Howting. "The Support Needs of Terminally Ill People Living Alone at Home: a Narrative Review." *Health Psychology and Behavioral Medicine* 2, no. 1 (2014): 951–69. https://doi.org/10.1080/21642850.2014.933342.

The need for earlier discussion of issues surrounding end-of-life care:

Khullar, Dhruv. "We're bad at death. Can we talk?" *New York Times,* May 10, 2017. https://www.nytimes.com/2017/05/10/upshot/were-bad-at-death-first-we-need-a-good-talk.html.

Prepare for our inevitable mortality:

Gerwig, A. "Why We Don't Talk about Death (but Should)." Legacy.com. October 1, 2015. http://www.legacy.com/news/advice-and-support/article/why-we-dont-talk-about-death-but-should

A disorienting fog of treatments and their side effects:

Myers, G. "Over-Medicalized Care at the End-of-Life in the United States." Turn-Key Health. December 2016. http://turn-keyhealth.com/wp-content/uploads/2016/12/Over-Medicalized-Care-at-the-End-of-Life-in-the-US.pdf.

Less than 15 percent of adults in the United States have one:

Alfonso, Heather. "The Importance of Living Wills and Advance Directives." *Journal of Gerontological Nursing* 35, no. 10 (2009): 42–45. https://doi.org/10.3928/00989134-20090903-05.

Efforts made by the medical team to back off on treatments, no matter how futile:

Wojtasiewicz, Mary Ellen. "Damage Compounded: Disparities, Distrust, and Disparate Impact in End-of-Life Conflict Resolution Policies." *The American Journal of Bioethics* 6, no. 5 (2006): 8–12. https://doi.org/10.1080/15265160600856801.

Open communication with families is imperative:

Fins, Joseph J. and Mildred Z. Solomon. "Communication in Intensive Care Settings: The Challenge of Futility Disputes." *Critical Care Medicine* 29, no. Supplement (2001). https://doi.org/10.1097/00003246-200102001-00003.

REFERENCES

African American patients more likely to die in the hospital than white patients:

Johnson, Kimberly S. "Racial and Ethnic Disparities in Palliative Care." *Journal of Palliative Medicine* 16, no. 11 (2013): 1329–34. https://doi.org/10.1089/jpm.2013.9468. See also Kwak, J., W. E. Haley, and D. A. Chiriboga. "Racial Differences in Hospice Use and In-Hospital Death among Medicare and Medicaid Dual-Eligible Nursing Home Residents." *The Gerontologist* 48, no. 1 (2008): 32–41. https://doi.org/10.1093/geront/48.1.32.

Transitioning to less intensive treatments:

Magarotto, Roberto, Gianluigi Lunardi, Francesca Coati, Paola Cassandrini, Vincenzo Picece, Silvia Ferrighi, Luciana Oliosi, and Marco Venturini. "Reduced Use of Chemotherapy at the End of Life in an Integrated-Care Model of Oncology and Palliative care. *Tumori*, 97, no. 5 (2011): 573–77. https://doi.org/10.1700/989.10714.

Medically appropriate decision-making:

Levine, Shanna R., Earle I. Bridget, and Wendy S.A. Edwards. "The Sooner the Better: Analysis of Proactive Palliative Medicine Consultation in the Medical Intensive Care Unit amongst Patients with Stage IV Malignancy." *Journal of Clinical Oncology* 32, no. 31_suppl (2014): 78–78. https://doi.org/10.1200/jco.2014.32.31_suppl.78.

Changing the name to "supportive care":

Dalal, Shalini, Shana Palla, David Hui, Linh Nguyen, Ray Chacko, Zhijun Li, Nada Fadul, Cheryl Scott, Veatra Thornton, and Brenda Coldman. "Association between a Name Change from Palliative to Supportive Care and the Timing of Patient Referrals at a Comprehensive Cancer Center." *The Oncologist* 16, no. 1 (2011): 105–11. https://doi.org/10.1634/theoncologist.2010-0161.

Pushing palliative care upstream into the clinic:

Blechman, Jennifer and Janet Bull. "Pushing Palliative Care Upstream: Integration into a Community-Based Oncology Practice." *Journal of Clinical Oncology* 33, no. 29_suppl (2015): 134. https://doi.org/10.1200/jco.2015.33.29_suppl.134.

Trained volunteers provide support to dying patients:

Corporon, Kathleen. "Comfort and Caring at the End of Life: Baylor's Doula Program." *Baylor University Medical Center Proceedings* 24, no. 4 (2011): 318–19. https://doi.org/10.1080/08998280.2011.11928748.

Typically referring only late in an illness:

Johnson, C.E., A. Girgis, C. Paul, and D. C. Currow. "Cancer Specialists' Palliative Care Referral Practices and Perceptions: Results of a National Survey." *Palliative Medicine* 22, no. 1 (2008): 51–57. https://doi.org/10.1177/0269216307085181.

No training in palliative care:

Griffin, Shannon, Juliette Cubanski, Tricia Neuman, Anne Jankiewicz, David Rousseau, and Kaiser Family Foundation. "Medicare and End-of-Life Care." *Jama* 316, no. 17 (2016): 1754. https://doi.org/10.1001/jama.2016.15577.

Who have been diagnosed with a serious illness:

Kelley, Amy S. and R. Sean Morrison. "Palliative Care for the Seriously Ill." *New England Journal of Medicine* 373, no. 8 (2015): 747–55. https://doi.org/10.1056/nejmra1404684.

Assist with complex medical decision-making, and coordination of care:

Kelley, Amy S. and R. Sean Morrison. "Palliative Care for the Seriously Ill." *New England Journal of Medicine* 373, no. 8 (2015): 747–55. https://doi.org/10.1056/nejmra1404684.

Still unevenly available in the United States:

Kelley, Amy S. and R. Sean Morrison. "Palliative Care for the Seriously Ill." *New England Journal of Medicine* 373, no. 8 (2015): 747–55. https://doi.org/10.1056/nejmra1404684.

Disparities based on socioeconomic and racial status of patients:

Dumanovsky, Tamara, Rachel Augustin, Maggie Rogers, Katrina Lettang, Diane E. Meier, and R. Sean Morrison. "The Growth of Palliative Care in U.S. Hospitals: A Status Report." *Journal of Palliative Medicine* 19, no. 1 (2016): 8–15. https://doi.org/10.1089/jpm.2015.0351.

See also Kwak, J., W. E. Haley, and D. A. Chiriboga. "Racial Differences in Hospice Use and In-Hospital Death among Medicare and Medicaid Dual-Eligible Nursing Home Residents." *The Gerontologist* 48, no. 1 (2008): 32–41.

Johnson, Kimberly S. "Racial and Ethnic Disparities in Palliative Care." *Journal of Palliative Medicine* 16, no. 11 (2013): 1329–34.

REFERENCES

Shortage of palliative care physicians across the United States:

Kelley, Amy S. and R. Sean Morrison. "Palliative Care for the Seriously Ill." *New England Journal of Medicine* 373, no. 8 (2015): 747–55. https://doi.org/10.1056/nejmra1404684.

More Americans are dying at home:

Kolata, Gina. "More Americans Are Dying at Home than in Hospitals." *New York Times.* December 11, 2019. https://www.nytimes.com/2019/12/11/health/death-hospitals-home.html.

Lags behind in these diagnoses:

Khullar, Dhruv. "We're bad at death. Can we talk?" *New York Times,* May 10, 2017. https://www.nytimes.com/2017/05/10/upshot/were-bad-at-death-first-we-need-a-good-talk.html.

A recently published article from Duke University:

Leblanc, Thomas W., Laura J. Fish, Catherine T. Bloom, Areej El-Jawahri, Debra M. Davis, Susan C. Locke, Karen E. Steinhauser, and Kathryn I. Pollak. "Patient Experiences of Acute Myeloid Leukemia: A Qualitative Study about Diagnosis, Illness Understanding, and Treatment Decision-Making." *Psycho-Oncology* 26, no. 12 (2016): 2063–68. https://doi.org/10.1002/pon.4309.

Ken Murray's "How Doctors Die":

Murray, K. "How Doctors Die." Zócalo Public Square. November 30, 2011. http://www.zocalopublicsquare.org/2011/11/30/how-doctors-die/ideas/nexus/.

Blecker, Saul, Norman J. Johnson, Sean Altekruse, and Leora I. Horwitz. "Association of Occupation as a Physician with Likelihood of Dying in a Hospital." *JAMA* 315, no. 3 (2016): 301. https://doi.org/10.1001/jama.2015.16976.

Earlier palliative care drives these down:

Morrison, R. Sean. "Cost Savings Associated With US Hospital Palliative Care Consultation Programs." *Archives of Internal Medicine* 168, no. 16 (2008): 1783. https://doi.org/10.1001/archinte.168.16.1783.

Speaking with patients and their families about end-of-life care:

Balaban, Richard B. "A Physician's Guide to Talking about End-of-Life Care." *Journal of General Internal Medicine* 15, no. 3 (2000): 195–200. https://doi.org/10.1046/j.1525-1497.2000.07228.x.

ADDITIONAL SOURCES

Dalal, Shalini and Eduardo Bruera. "End-of-Life Care Matters: Palliative Cancer Care Results in Better Care and Lower Costs." *The Oncologist* 22, no. 4 (2017): 361–68. https://doi.org/10.1634/theoncologist.2016-0277.

Frontera, Jennifer A., J. Randall Curtis, Judith E. Nelson, Margaret Campbell, Michelle Gabriel, Anne C. Mosenthal, Colleen Mulkerin, Kathleen A. Puntillo, Daniel E. Ray, and Rick Bassett. "Integrating Palliative Care into the Care of Neurocritically Ill Patients." *Critical Care Medicine* 43, no. 9 (2015): 1964–77. https://doi.org/10.1097/ccm.0000000000001131.

Mackintosh, David. "Death as 'Harm' When It Is an Anticipated Outcome in Palliative Care—Or Anywhere." *Journal of Palliative Medicine* 17, no. 5 (2014): 502. https://doi.org/10.1089/jpm.2014.0018.

Mar, JoAnn. "Racial Disparities in End-of-Life Care: How Mistrust Keeps Many African-Americans Away from Hospice." KALW. November 14, 2018. https://www.kalw.org/post/racial-disparities-end-life-care-how-mistrust-keeps-many-african-americans-away-hospice.

Papadopoulou, Constantina, Bridget Johnston, and Markus Themessl-Huber. "The Experience of Acute Leukaemia in Adult Patients: A Qualitative Thematic Synthesis." *European Journal of Oncology Nursing* 17, no. 5 (2013): 640–48. https://doi.org/10.1016/j.ejon.2013.06.009.

Ruddy, Kathryn J., Betsy C. Risendal, Judy E. Garber, and Ann H. Partridge. "Cancer Survivorship Care: An Opportunity to Revisit Cancer Genetics." *Journal of Clinical Oncology* 34, no. 6 (2016): 539–41. https://doi.org/10.1200/jco.2015.63.5375.

Shapiro, Susan P. *Speaking for the Dying: Life-and Death Decisions in Intensive Care.* Chicago, IL: The University of Chicago Press, 2019.

Yanada, Masamitsu, Akinao Okamoto, Yoko Inaguma, Masutaka Tokuda, Satoko Morishima, Tadaharu Kanie, Yukiya Yamamoto, Shuichi Mizuta, Yoshiki Akatsuka, Masataka Okamoto et al. "The Fate of Patients with Acute Myeloid Leukemia not Undergoing Induction Chemotherapy." *International Journal of Hematology* 102, no. 1 (2015): 35–40. https://doi.org/10.1007/s12185-015-1786-0.

CHAPTER TWELVE: COMPASSION AS A CORE VALUE

Approximately 55 percent of physicians admit to being burned out:

Drummond, Dike. *Stop Physician Burnout: What To Do When Working Harder Isn't Working.* New York: Heritage Press Publications, 2014.

Depending on the severity of this experience:

Maslach, Chrostina, Susan Jackson, and Michael Leiter. *Maslach Burnout Inventory Manual*. Palo Alto, California: Consulting Psychological Press, Inc., 1996.

"Compassion fatigue":

Peckham, C. "Medscape Lifestyle Report 2017: Race and Ethnicity, Bias and Burnout," Medscape (2017) 1–28. http://www.medscape.com/features/slideshow/lifestyle/2017/overview.

Inability to process grief and loss personally and within our professional lives:

Granek, Leeat, Merav Ben-David, Ora Nakash, Michal Cohen, Lisa Barbera, Samuel Ariad, and Monika K. Krzyzanowska. "Oncologists' Negative Attitudes towards Expressing Emotion over Patient Death and Burnout." *Supportive Care in Cancer* 25, no. 5 (2017): 1607–14. https://doi.org/10.1007/s00520-016-3562-y.

See also Kalra, Jagmohan, Fred Rosner, and Stanley Shapiro. "Emotional Strain on Physicians Caring for Cancer Patients. *Loss, Grief & Care*, no 1 (1987): 3–4, 19–24.

Pfifferling, John Henry and Kay Gilley. "Overcoming Compassion Fatigue." *Family Practice Management*, 7, no. 4 (2000): 39.

Discuss their failures and sadness:

Granek, Leeat, Merav Ben-David, Ora Nakash, Michal Cohen, Lisa Barbera, Samuel Ariad, and Monika K. Krzyzanowska. "Oncologists' Negative Attitudes towards Expressing Emotion over Patient Death and Burnout." *Supportive Care in Cancer* 25, no. 5 (2017): 1607–14. https://doi.org/10.1007/s00520-016-3562-y.

Doctors do so at their own risk:

Drummond, Dike. *Stop Physician Burnout: What To Do When Working Harder Isn't Working*. New York: Heritage Press Publications, 2014.

Improve the patient experience and maintain dignity in the ICU:

Cook, Deborah and Graeme Rocker. "Dying with Dignity in the Intensive Care Unit." *New England Journal of Medicine* 370, no. 26 (2014): 2506–14. https://doi.org/10.1056/nejmra1208795.

See also Carrese, Joseph, Lindsay Forbes, Emily Branyon, Hanan Aboumatar, Gail Geller, Mary Catherine Beach, and Jeremy Sugarman. "Observations of Respect and Dignity in the Intensive Care Unit." *Narrative Inquiry in Bioethics* 5, no. 1A (2015). https://doi.org/10.1353/nib.2015.0002.

The sleep deprivation that is a hallmark of a stay in the ICU:

Beltrami, Flávia Gabe, Xuân-Lan Nguyen, Claire Pichereau, Eric Maury, Bernard Fleury, and Simone Fagondes. "Sleep in the Intensive Care Unit." *Jornal Brasileiro de Pneumologia* 41, no. 6 (2015): 539–46. https://doi.org/10.1590/s1806-37562015000000056.

See also Delves, Jillian. "Sleep Deprivation in the Intensive Care Unit." *HNE Handover: For Nurses and Midwives*, 2, no. 1 (2009). Accessed at http://journals.sfu.ca/hneh/index.php/hneh/article/view/48.

Durrington, Hannah J., Richard Clark, Ruari Greer, Franck P. Martial, John Blaikley, Paul Dark, Robert J. Lucas, and David W. Ray. "'In a Dark Place, We Find Ourselves': Light Intensity in Critical Care Units." *Intensive Care Medicine Experimental* 5, no. 1 (2017). https://doi.org/10.1186/s40635-017-0122-9.

Oldham, Mark A., Hochang B. Lee, and Paul H. Desan. "Circadian Rhythm Disruption in the Critically Ill." *Critical Care Medicine* 44, no. 1 (2016): 207–17. https://doi.org/10.1097/ccm.0000000000001282.

Weinhouse, Gerald L. and Richard J. Schwab. "Sleep in the Critically Ill Patient." *Sleep*, 29, no. 5 (2006): 707–16.

Appropriate for maintaining a restful environment:

Weinhouse, Gerald L. and Richard J. Schwab. "Sleep in the Critically Ill Patient." *Sleep*, 29, no. 5 (2006): 707–16.

Out of regard for the patients:

Beltrami, Flávia Gabe, Xuân-Lan Nguyen, Claire Pichereau, Eric Maury, Bernard Fleury, and Simone Fagondes. "Sleep in the Intensive Care Unit." *Jornal Brasileiro de Pneumologia* 41, no. 6 (2015): 539–46. https://doi.org/10.1590/s1806-37562015000000056.

ADDITIONAL SOURCES

Halpern, Jodi. *From Detached Concern to Empathy: Humanizing Medical Practice*. Oxford: Oxford University Press, 2001.

Trzeciak, Stephen and Anthony Mazzarelli. *Compassionomics: The Revolutionary Scientific Evidence That Caring Makes a Difference*. Pensacola, FL: Studer Group Publishing, 2019.

CONCLUSION: COMPASSION AND CORONAVIRUS

Suicide of Dr. Lorna Breen:

Watkins, Ali, William K Rashbaum, and Brian M.Rosenthal. "Top E.R. Doctor Who Treated Virus Patients Dies By Suicide." *New York Times*, April 27, 2020. https://www.nytimes.com/2020/04/27/nyregion/new-york-city-doctor-suicide-coronavirus.html.

EPIGRAPH SOURCES

Kenyon, Jane. "Prognosis" and "Chrysanthemums." In *Otherwise*. St. Paul, MN: Graywolf Press, 1997.

Kristof, Nicholas. "Life and Death in the 'Hot Zone.'" *New York Times*, April 12, 2020. https://www.nytimes.com/2020/04/11/opinion/sunday/coronavirus-hospitals-bronx.html.

Miller, BJ, "What Really Matters at the End of Life," filmed March 2015 at TED2015: Truth and Dare, Vancouver, BC. Video, 19:07. https://www.youtube.com/watch?v=apbSsILLh28&t=285s.

Mother Teresa quote. In Paul, Kimberly C. *Bridging the Gap: Life Lessons from the Dying*. Pennsauken, NJ: BookBaby, 2018.

Oliver, Mary. "The Wind in the Pines." In *Swan: Poems and Prose Poems*. Boston: Beacon Press, 2010.

Snicket, Lemony. *Horseradish: Bitter Truths You Can't Avoid*. New York: HarperCollins, 2007.

Trzeciak, Stephen and Anthony Mazzarelli. *Compassionomics: The Revolutionary Scientific Evidence That Caring Makes a Difference*. Pensacola, FL: Studer Group Publishing, 2019.

Wilder, Thornton. *Our Town: A Play in Three Acts*. New York: Harper Perennial, 2003.